THE PATIENT'S VOICE:

Experiences of Illness

THE PATIENT'S VOICE:
Experiences of Illness

Jeanine Young-Mason, EdD, RN, CS, FAAN
Associate Professor, School of Nursing,
University of Massachusetts at Amherst, Amherst, MA

 F. A. DAVIS COMPANY • Philadelphia

F. A. Davis Company
1915 Arch Street
Philadelphia, PA 19103

Printed in the United States of America

Last digit indicates print number: 10 9 8 7 6 5 4

Publisher, Nursing: Robert G. Martone
Nursing Developmental Editor: Joanne P. DaCunha, RN, MSN
Production Editor: Roberta Massey
Cover Designer: Steven Ross Morrone

As new scientific information becomes available through basic and clinical research, recom-mended treatments and drug therapies undergo changes. The author and publisher have done everything possible to make this book accurate, up to date, and in accord with accepted standards at the time of publication. The author, editors, and publisher are not responsible for errors or omissions or for consequences from application of the book, and make no warranty, expressed or implied, in regard to the contents of the book. Any practice described in this book should be applied by the reader in accordance with professional standards of care used in regard to the unique circumstances that may apply in each situation. The reader is advised always to check product information (package inserts) for changes and new information regarding dose and con-traindications before administering any drug. Caution is especially urged when using new or infrequently ordered drugs.

Library of Congress Cataloging-in-Publication Data

The patient's voice: experiences of illness/[edited by] Jeanine Young-Mason.
    p. cm.
   ISBN 0-8036-0162-X (alk. paper)
    1. Sick—Psychology.   2. Sick—Attitudes.   3. Health attitudes.   4. Sick—Interviews.
I. Young-Mason, Jeanine, 1938-
   [DNLM: 1. Patients—psychology. 2. Attitude to Health. 3. Mental Disorders—psy-chology. W 85 P29888   1997]
   R726.5.P375   1997
   155.9' 16—dc20
   DNLM/DLC
   for Library of Congress   96-28901

Dedicated with deep gratitude to the authors of these narratives for sharing their most private thoughts and experiences for our enrichment and learning and to Dino Cavallari For Painting "Le Voix du Malade" expressly for this book.

With sincere appreciation for Joanne DaCunha and Jane Carter for their role in making this book's publication possible and to Peter Faber for his careful supervision of its production.

Preface

———— ∎ ————

The *Patient's Voice: Experiences of Illness* introduces contemporary autobiographical accounts of psychiatric and somatic illness to students in nursing, medicine, and allied health professions. The accounts, written expressly for this book, are of children's and adults' experiences of illness. They emphasize the implications of illness and spiritual distress and the ways in which the individuals express their views of compassionate care.

The contributors write with authenticity and courage about their lived experiences and in so doing offer to students of the human condition a unique body of information not ordinarily available in textbooks. This information is both insightful and pragmatic and has the potential to enlighten and enrich the practitioner's personal and professional life. Each account teaches the student something about the experience of illness and loss and deepens our understanding of suffering and the restorative power of compassion. Furthermore, the accounts instruct us on how to deal practically and politically with such conditions in contexts in which individuals find themselves disadvantaged and vulnerable.

These contributors, known personally to the author, are by profession health care providers, lawyers, students, teachers, and writers known for their writing ability and the quality of their perceptions.

The book's 16 accounts are arranged according to the breadth of life, beginning with accounts of and about children and ending with those of adults. Each chapter ends with points for discussion and writing intended to assist students in learning how to interpret and understand the individual's account. These points were devised by the author and the contributors to the book.

Contents

I know that sorrow is private and inward, even if in some sense ritually shared and partially diffused. I have learned over the years that loss can be transformed through grief into a personal ideology of distrust, exclusiveness, and even hate. In defiance of this, however, it is also possible, through compassion and not just ordinary understanding, to reach a gradual convalescence and an end to death's deforming of ourselves.

Herbert Mason

After nearly 35 years, my relationship with muscular dystrophy, like any other long-term relationship, has grown exceedingly close and complex. We have forged a bond as fellow travelers, and traveling the road together has taught me to fight but also to cherish life and the people who give that life meaning. For a long time I believed that the disease could not be real if I refused to acknowledge its existence—if I kept it out of sight. But I have always known my disease-companion to be close by, waiting just beyond my vision. Now I find that I prefer to invite my companion into the light of the fire rather than search for his eyes in the dark.

Allan H. Macurdy

I remember the years of trying to teach him to throw a ball at all and marvel at his accomplishments. I'm left with some of my own dearest memories, like putting Raoul to bed, closing the door, and hearing "Mom?" "Yes, Raoul?" "What if the bus doesn't come?" "Don't worry, it will come in the morning. Go to sleep." "Mom?" "Don't worry, I love you."

Dorothy C. Buck

When something is painful or boring you never forget it. I think I remember all this stuff because they were both. I also mention friends a lot because friends play a huge role in my recovery.

Gertrude Simpson

sincere in her concern, truly compassionate, and caring, simply because she was direct and had her own problems.

That, I think, unites those who share this planet. Suffering is everywhere, and when one has passed through that cauldron, a sincere hand and heart survive in the mind as the warmest of memories. Be interested in people, their lives and their families. It is vital that you not feel like a total patient. Hell, we're all patients in this universe we share now.

Gene Higgins

I don't think anyone has an answer. It is as if it is too new or an unexplored area. Is it an emotional problem brought on by disease, resentment, the end of the marriage in real sharing terms, or simply the inability to deal with any or all of these things?

I don't know the answer and neither do the doctors thus far. However, they should try to recognize the unhappiness factor and understand its effect on one's physical and emotional state.

James Armstrong

If we focus on the victim and not on where the money is coming from, then we want to go on doing our dance until the victim is made "well" and our own prosperity is thereby increased.

Mark Maclean Rufo

. . . Sharing pain is the only way to stay alive. For the net of love helps absorb and distribute the struggle. It's taught me that if we share pain, which is a lot to ask, there is no room for pity. For the sharing of the struggle requires an investment, a real life-changing investment by those who care, an involvement that will instigate their own tandem suffering.

Mark Nepo

Suffering may be an opportunity to face a deeper part of ourselves, a part we all must face sooner or later since we are all mortal. And that suffering may be necessary for our transformation, to help us realize, in the sense of "making real," a more profound, inner experience of life. In this we may be assisting the interpenetration of higher and lower, truly bringing the sacred into our lives.

Rebecca Sachs Norris

So often, people would comment on how wonderful it was that I cared for and was with my friend through her dying and give me undue praise and acknowledgement. But it is I who feel humbled to have been allowed by my friend to share in such an intimate and personal experience, which would ultimately change my life forever, and it is I who am grateful for what she gave me.

Linda Q. Trott

The Memory of Death

Herbert Mason

Herbert Mason is University Professor of History and Religion at Boston University, specializing in Islamic and Near Eastern Studies. He is the author of 13 books, including his National Book Award nominee *Gilgamesh: a Verse Narrative*, and his most recent *al-Hallaj*, an interpretive history of a 10th-century Muslim mystic. In addition to his historical works and his translations from Arabic and French, he has published fiction and poetry.

In 1939, when Herbert Mason was 7 years old, his father died suddenly and unexpectedly. His vivid memories of that fateful day and its penetrating effects and influences upon his life and life's work offer important insights into the workings of grief.

The Memory of Death

by Herbert Mason

It is that inner atmosphere that has
An unfamiliar gravity or none at all
Where words are flung out in the air but stay
Motionless without an answer,
Hovering about one's lips
Or arguing back to haunt
The memory with what one failed to say,
Until one learns acceptance of the silence
Amidst the new debris
Or turns again to grief
As the only source of privacy,
Alone with someone loved.
It could go on for years and years,
And has, for centuries,
For being human holds a special grief
Of privacy within the universe
That yearns and waits to be retouched
By someone who can take away
The memory of death.

Herbert Mason, *Gilgamesh: a Verse Narrative*

*B*ecause the power of death yields in some of us such a longevity of grief, it is surely appropriate to include it among chronicles of illness. Indeed, grief, on a personal and collective scale, may be the most all-consuming, inescapable, and indecipherable of all illnesses suffered by humanity. I learned as a child of 7 at my father's death that grief is shared with others and others' tears can drown out one's own to the point where one can't hear oneself or be heard. We are made suddenly fearful. And for those of us who view death as a tragedy, whether we laugh at it like the Irish of old or quietly weep like the ancient Mesopotamians with their distended eyes, it causes terror, such that only very gradually over time, over years, are we brought to rise up in frail but humanly heroic defiance of death's power. Before heroism rises in us, this fearfulness results in some of the strangest, most bewildering behavior that human beings are capable of, much of it rooted in our competitiveness, possessiveness, and capacity for jealousy.

The nurse, the widowed Mrs. Shanks, announced my father's death as a fact to all of us in our house in New Hampshire. First she told my sister and me alone in my parents' bedroom upstairs. Then, after she left us two with this information, she went downstairs to announce it to my father's brother and his three children. The shrieks accompanied her from upstairs down and then flowed back to us up the stairway, like water swirling and rising in a flood. My sister and I, my three cousins, my uncle, and the nurse, who doubled as our cook and now caretaker, all of us went off alone in different directions, directionless. Only my uncle, who was mostly immobilized by his prior loss of sight, stayed in the music room where he was given the news, but stood up reaching out for a wall to hold onto. It was my first image through my tears as I passed the open door into the music room on my way outside where I would also be alone.

It was shared grief, grief filled with others' tears that drowned out my own, so I couldn't hear myself. I think this is why I banged the tall oak tree by the front door with my fists until they bled, demanding that I and my grief be heard, at least by me! I wanted my father, now above all times, to be mine alone. But so did everyone else. I had no way of knowing then how central my father had been to all their lives, his brother's, my cousins. I didn't know that he had paid for this one's violin lessons, that one's schooling, this one's orthodontia, their mother's hospital bills when his brother's retirement fund and inheritance ran out. I only knew that a week before he died, when he was with us in New Hampshire, my cousin Bert, then 16, had wrecked our car driving down the valley to Alstead. When a farmer passing by the wreck picked him up, bruised but mainly ashamed, and brought him back up to us, my father put his arms around him as he wept. I wanted those arms myself, then, when he was gone.

When my older sister and I first saw our mother after we learned from the nurse of our father's death, her face was scarlet, a deeper color than her usual long red hair. She was dressed in black, wore dark glasses, which she removed when she approached us. She shocked us even further, virtually out of our own grief, when we saw the devastation in her eyes. For years after, we each felt a strange priority, a deep entitlement, to our separate griefs and could barely speak to each other, let alone to others, about our innermost possession of grief. In a sense death separated us permanently as members of a family.

After our father's funeral—my sister and I were not taken to the cemetery but remained at home with the nurse and caterers for the reception that followed—I was swept aside yet again by the wails and stares of my father's many relatives, friends, and coworkers, all of whom were just so many strangers. A convergence of two things still remains most remarkable about the sudden moment of solitude in which I found myself.

The first was the vivid and deep sense of my father's presence in the living room where I was left alone. By this I mean his physical presence. Though I couldn't see him,

I knew he was there and looked for him first behind the long curtains hanging down beside the tall windows. When I realized he wasn't merely hiding but was truly there, I stopped looking in actual places and stood still, sensing him everywhere. He remained with me in that sense beyond that day, indeed for years. It was in fact something I couldn't speak about to anyone, and for that reason it was isolating, inhibiting, retarding my social and academic life. At times it became like a scar or birthmark that I covered with my hand lest someone see and mock it. The scar wasn't the fact of being fatherless, and thus unlike others I knew in school. Rather it was a separate companionship, a fantasy more real than living people. I think I believed my father and I were two disembodied spirits who had left the human world forever, together as one. My long-range problem was coming back, inevitably, to the human world, where death dictated and its hell of griefs reigned supreme.

(When I was 12, I was mysteriously ill for an entire year. No clear explanation emerged from any of the doctors my mother took me to. One day I overheard one of my father's closest friends tell my mother it was "heart sickness," meaning a broken heart. "He loved his father too intensely.")

My sister, who was 12 when my father died, was more socialized than I and immersed herself in serious friendships, one of the most restorative of all immersions. My mother, however, 3 days after the funeral screamed, "Nothing is there! Nothing there!" and threw herself down the attic stairs in the first of many desperate attempts and countless threats to kill herself in those early years. The result of her flight was a few days in the hospital and a broken arm set at a permanent right angle at the elbow by the same local doctor who had misdiagnosed my father after his automobile accident. The doctor didn't suspect from the blood in his eyes and deep discoloration of his forehead any hint of the cerebral hemorrhage that killed him within a week.

The second, even stranger presence in the living room that day of the funeral was the appearance of my uncle's daughter, my cousin Louisa, who I was told much later was schizophrenic, and was eventually, sadly, institutionalized.

We were left briefly together in the living room, unwittingly placed together, away from the interment; she was deeply fond of my father and might have acted strangely, whereas I was simply judged too young to go. To me, then, Louisa was even sadder than myself. She put her cheek against the cabinet of our radio with the volume as high as it could go, and she stared at me while she beat the cabinet with her fingers as if it were her dead mother's cello. I was scared and yet I was also strangely reassured by my father's presence there with us, a presence that was always kind and embracing. At one moment, in fact, she looked at me very closely and very sadly, and without either of us speaking, she turned the volume down. My father seemed to have enfolded both of us in his arms and let us be ourselves in that brief moment together.

My mother, who lived into her 96th year and was ultimately interred in the same cemetery as my father in December 1991, had a very different and quite renewing later life. Eventually, she, my sister, and I released each other from our lives that had long ago been separated by loss. My mother gave copies of my retelling of the old Babylonian epic of *Gilgamesh* to relatives and friends, but I don't believe she read it, for she once said to me when she was 80 and still in command of her powers of mind and body that she "understood," as she put it, "that it was very painful to read," and she didn't want "to relive the pain."

To deal fully with the isolation and, more important, the longevity of grief that began for me with my father's sudden and unexpected death, I have gradually found some understanding of the "illness" as an adult faced with my own mortality and that of other loved ones lost. As I recollect today my experience as a child of 7 who had just lost to death the one he most loved in this world—a child who was literally lost in a swirl of unwanted convergences, when his only constant guide and companion was pain, I know that sorrow is private and inward, even if in some sense ritually shared and partially diffused. I have learned over the years that loss can be transformed through grief into a personal ideology of distrust, exclusiveness, and even hate. In defiance of this, however, it is also possible, through compassion and not just ordinary understanding, to reach a gradual convalescence and an end to death's deformation of ourselves.

■

I would suggest a few things as possible flash points that might be helpful in understanding those in grieving states.

First, grief puts a person in a state of deep isolation, sometimes for a long time. Further, grief makes one very possessive and self-centered and competitive with others who were close to the deceased. For a time, then, one who grieves may try to identify with other sufferers, expecting to receive understanding. Eventually, however, one resents being included, as one is among the pariahs of society, and withdraws into even deeper solitude. Grieving doesn't necessarily sensitize anyone and often it only desensitizes and isolates. To some the loved one who is deceased becomes the only recourse in a private world from which others without the same knowledge are excluded. Though there is always a desire to be understood and treated kindly, in grief one may lose the ability to inspire such responses.

Grief, which is a spiritual illness derived from a loved one's death, has physical effects that cannot be diagnosed and treated simply. The impact is sudden. One's healing responses are unprepared and thwarted, and the expectation of recovery is indeterminate. For some, such a spiritual initiative, a so-called act of God, may lead to a religious quest, and even a conversion, but for others, it can result in the reverse, in spiritual despair of any promise of redemption and of humanity's capacity for giving or meriting compassion. It isn't certain which state will befall us individually: Whether we come from a religious or a skeptical tradition, neither can prepare us for the loss of a loved one and both share ignorance at death.

We learn from a loved one's death, most of all, that our deepest yearning for ourselves and all humanity is for that transcendent that compassion that can only come from the source that also gives life. And from that yearning and that compassion working in and through us can come a wisdom that enables us to resume living.

CRITICAL-THINKING ACTIVITIES

1. Explain the reasons why grief isolates the members of this family.

2. How is the mother's grief and despair manifested? Describe its effects on the author.

3. Explain the author's experience of his father's presence in the room with him the day of the funeral.

4. What happened to the narrator when he became mysteriously ill at age 12? How was this illness affected by grief?

5. How is the author's experience of grief distilled in the lines from *Gilgamesh*?

6. How do the members of this family compete with one another in grief? Explain and discuss.

7. Delineate and discuss Professor Mason's flash points in the experience of grief, using examples from the narrative.

8. Write a study of a young child who has experienced the loss of a parent. Compare this child's experience with that of Professor Mason.

9. Should young children be excluded from funerals and interments? Defend your answer.

10. Discuss in detail a childhood experience of grief that taught you something important about loss.

Allan H. Macurdy

Allan H. Macurdy is a lecturer in law at Boston University School of Law, a staff attorney at Pike Institute on Law and Disability, and an adjunct professor of law at Boston College, Northeastern University and New England School of Law. He earned his JD at Boston University School of Law and his BA in history at Boston University.

When Allan H. Macurdy was 8 years old he and his parents were told that he had muscular dystrophy, which would lead to his "demise, probably by the age of 15." Despite the presence and progression of the disease, Macurdy is now a practicing lawyer in his mid-thirties who lives with his wife and dog and teaches law students full-time. Through his experiences with his "disease-companion" and the politics of health care, he has fashioned four principles that govern his interactions with health-care professionals and the medical system and track, to a great extent, the manner in which he conducts his life as an individual with a disability.

CHAPTER 2

Mastery of Life

by Allan H. Macurdy

Muscular dystrophy and I are lifelong companions, and though I know our mortal enmity will some day be tested (and I will lose), we have maintained a relationship of wary coexistence. The disease and I were first introduced in second grade when I was diagnosed, but we had been intimately connected from the moment my parents conceived me, their eldest son. As a genetic disorder, muscular dystrophy is as much a part of my identity as my eye color, my height, or my resemblance to my parents. It was never an invader: the disease and I have fought for control over territory to which we both felt entitled.

Our introduction took the form of a death sentence, albeit in clinical language. When I was 8 years old my parents were told that I had the disease and that it would lead to my demise, probably by age 15. Oblivious to the positivist echoes attached to the word, the medical community describes Duchenne's muscular dystrophy as a "progressive" disorder, meaning only that the disease continues to destroy muscle tissue until it kills you. First, I would lose the voluntary muscles that enabled me to use my arms and legs. Then the muscles in the abdomen that permitted standing or sitting without support would fail. Finally, the disease would move on to my respiratory and cardiac muscles and I would die. However devastating to my parents, all this was beyond my understanding as an 8-year-old, but at least there was now an answer when I asked why I fell down a lot or why I walked funny.

During my childhood, I rarely saw my disease-companion sitting at my table, and even more rarely thought about the role the disease played, and was to play, in my life. Such dark thoughts were not a feature of my happy childhood. Indeed, I lived the typical life of a small boy in suburbia, full of tree forts, puppies, and baseball. Friends were everything, did everything. We pretended we were superheroes or professional athletes. We delighted in mischief. We disliked girls intensely. But muscular dystrophy was involved in much of my life and determined that my experiences would be atypical.

At age 8 or 9, when my friends would play in the school yard, I began to notice that I couldn't keep up with the other kids. I was always last in races and was frequently tagged out, as were many kids, but it seemed that I never had enough energy for play. My most hated activity was the long climb to the second floor for art class. Each step in the flight was a new battle to get both feet on the next step while hanging on to the banister for support. But I also had classmates who were terrible at sports or winded by that same flight of stairs.

It was my experiences with the medical system, however, that most clearly differed from anything in my friends' lives. Although I was examined by many different doctors in my parents' effort to have my condition diagnosed, my earliest memory of hospitals and doctors came during second grade, when I spent a week in Riverview Hospital undergoing tests. Having been to school, I knew I didn't like tests, but these were so strange that I almost began to enjoy them. In one room, some man glued wires to my head, dimmed the lights, and told me to think about a rabbit. In another room, a beautiful lady took a scary needle and put it in my leg, but it didn't hurt. Because these people were friendly and took the time to explain what was happening and why, this was not a terrifying experience.

After the doctors determined that I did indeed have muscular dystrophy, I encountered the health-care world in brief visits with various professionals. I saw my orthopedist and the physical therapist on a monthly basis, with occasional trips to the brace maker or hospital x-ray department. But my battle with the disease at this stage of my life was fought largely apart from doctors and therapists. After all, they were focused upon slowing the inevitable march of deterioration, rather than the day-to-day realities of trying to be a kid. Not that our goals were in conflict: Inactivity would not only be intolerable for a child, but it would also accelerate the destruction of muscle tissue. So with the blessing of the medical world, the challenge of climbing the stairs to my bedroom or rising to my feet after a fall were the tangible victories I sought, and savored.

By adolescence, however, my weakened muscles could no longer support the efforts of my growing body. I could no longer climb those stairs, and if I fell, I was now required to wait until someone came along to help. To a teenager, reliance upon other people, particularly adults, is the perpetuation of childhood. From this perspective, to be an adult is to have achieved the perfection of independence. Anything that restricts any desire that a teen might have is perceived as an injustice, an effort to prevent entrance into adult privilege. For most teens, the source of those restrictions, and therefore those injustices, is their parents. But for me, the disease played that role: In fact, it was the inevitability that muscular dystrophy would prevent me from achieving the independence I so desperately wanted that bothered me the most. I had never really thought about it before, but at 13, I realized that I would probably be dead in 2 years. In the face of that reality, all my struggle against the disease seemed futile. And what could be more unjust?

For a time, my anger and frustration threatened to overwhelm me. That sense of powerlessness pervaded my inner self, and though time moved on, to me it appeared that I would never get beyond my rage. But I soon tired of the melodrama and began to get on with my life. For some reason, as I neared the end of junior high school, I was no longer so angry, no longer caught up in the futility of fighting the disease. More and more, I was seeing that there were more reasons to fight than to give up. I cannot point to any crystallizing moment when I found a purpose for my life or came to value the people around me. All I know, and all my parents knew, is that by this point I had gained faith that my life had value, and, for this reason, I was much easier to deal with. I was now able to concentrate on both being a kid and developing the social techniques to work around others' reactions to my disability.

Over the next decade, my life proceeded in much the same way as did the lives of my peers. I went to college, graduated, went on to law school, and prepared to enter my profession. Because the disease created only orthopedic problems, I learned to compensate for my physical limitations so effectively that the disease was nearly irrelevant.

But this seeming irrelevance was an illusion of my own making, not a permanent reality. The disease, my lifelong companion, was still very much with me. In the midst of bar exams and job searches, my respiratory system began to fail; the disease had destroyed enough of the muscles that enable me to breathe that I was no longer able to function effectively. As my breathing capacity diminished, the carbon dioxide in my bloodstream reached toxic levels. This led to a significant loss of stamina and concentration. In addition, because I couldn't expand my lungs I had frequent respiratory infections and pneumonias. I was no longer able to compensate for all these physical problems. This marked the beginning of an 18-month decline that increasingly forced me to seek out and rely upon medical professionals and the medical system.

In February 1987, 2 days before I was to sit for the bar examination, the chest cold I had been fighting deteriorated into a full-blown lower-respiratory infection. This was not unprecedented since, at age 27, I had certainly had my share of illness. But something about this infection was new and alarming. For the first time, I was unable to clear secretions from my airway by coughing and I was becoming increasingly short of breath. Chest x-rays confirmed Dr. Hill's suspicions of pneumonia. I was started on a course of antibiotics and chest physical therapy, but after 2 days in the hospital it became apparent that I would need some form of mechanical breathing assistance, at least until I had fought off the infection.

What happened then is a parable on the failings of the medical model to consider the person behind the symptoms. In treating respiratory failure brought on by muscular dystrophy, Dr. Hill had begun using the iron lung, a device long associated with the polio epidemic of the 1950s. I had a vague memory of seeing an old photograph of an iron lung in a book, but I was totally unprepared for the realities of using one—or the fear. Someone wheeled this huge steel cylinder with a mechanical bellows at one end into my room. Behind it, much like infantrymen advancing behind the cover of a Sherman tank, came a squad of residents and medical students chattering about test results and pressure settings. With little more than a passing acknowledgment that I existed, the resident in charge ordered the nurses to put me into the iron lung and began to quiz his squad on the technical minutiae of *my* case.

Pause for a moment to consider the situation I faced. There I was in this intensive care unit, fevered, my lungs full of secretions, and unable to get enough air. Such circumstances are frightening enough by themselves. In the midst of all that activity, my anxiety was heightened by the fact that no one was listening to me, no one seemed to be aware that I existed beyond the data in my chart. But more terrifying still was the iron lung, and the procedure necessary to being placed inside. First, the cylinder was opened and I was laid down completely flat inside, a position that made breathing even more difficult for me. Next, I was slid up so that my head passed through a hole in the end of the cylinder and rested on a shelf outside. I lay face up with a 3-foot steel ring around my neck like some grotesque Elizabethan ruff, unable to move my head more than half an inch in any direction.

All of this alone was enough to induce claustrophobia, but add an inability to breathe, carbon dioxide toxicity, and fever, and the result was abject terror. None of the residents seemed to notice, however. At a time when the right words could have allayed my fear, or at least pushed it back, instead I met words that trivialized and excluded. The residents chattered on among themselves with great enthusiasm about arterial blood gas levels, titer volumes, and the comparative advantages of negative versus positive pressure ventilation. But direct interaction with me consisted of awkward, perfunctory monologues, delivered with impatience and never followed by listening. Because stress makes breathing much more difficult, respiratory patients cannot fully benefit from treatment without controlling their emotions. I needed both information and the assurance that I would not be sacrificed to some other agenda, even when I could not devote breath to speech. My questions, and forthright answers, were central to my ability to cope with the anxiety of this crisis.

That the residents were completely lacking in respect or empathy was not only clear to me but also angered the nurses. Once the decision to put me into the iron lung had been made, the nurse assigned to my case—call him John—had to get me inside while dealing with my anxiety. John tried to explain what was to occur, and to offer calm reassurance, but each time he finished readying me for the process, the residents would transform my room into a noisy, chaotic disaster and he had to begin again. After the second false start, John asked the residents, quite nicely, if they would mind taking their discussion out of the room. They complied with his request, but their compliance was short-lived.

Finally John had had enough. Raising his voice above the din he said, "If you aren't going to help, get the hell out of here! You're making this ten times harder on Allan." The residents were instantly aroused to righteous indignation, but nonetheless they filed back out. Once they were gone for good, we succeeded in getting me from the bed into the lung. The cylinder was closed, a seal was made at my neck, and the bellows went into action. I had never before experienced that sense of total helplessness and vulnerability, and it was primarily the result of the residents' (and many other health professionals') failure to treat me as the decision maker, the most interested party, and an individual whose feelings counted. For all the attention they paid, I could easily not have even been in the room. I vowed never again to be marginalized by medical personnel.

In that hospital experience I learned many things about the medical system that had nothing to do with treating disease or caring, but everything to do with power. This system, like any other human system, is made up of political phenomena: hierarchies of professionals, chains of command, patterns of authority, institutional agendas. Seen as such, it no longer seems alien. Indeed, I have a political mind, so the system plays directly to my strength. Legally, all legitimate power is vested in the patient, providing, of course, that he or she is mentally competent and conscious. I was clearly both, but power will not tolerate a vacuum, so if I failed to use my power, someone else would. The device best suited to enhance the power of health professionals is their virtual monopoly on medical knowledge. Lack of access to information, except through such a professional, is extremely intimidating and causes the patient to give up a great deal of power. The institutions also coerce the patient through the loss of both privacy and scheduling autonomy.

Even the everyday language is laden with authoritarian nuance. If I as a patient were to decide, for any reason, not to take a given medication I would be described as "refusing" treatment, not "making a decision." If I were asked if I were in pain and answered in the negative, I would be "denying" pain, as if the pain exists but I just will not admit it. And if I were to "deny" or "refuse" too often, I would be labeled "noncompliant" with the supposedly legitimate authority of the medical professional. These few examples are indicative of at least a habit of mind, if not a system of belief, that regards patients as, at best, children in need of parental figures to make decisions for them, and confers superior status on the practitioner.

To be sure, most health professionals do not view their relationships with patients in such terms. Quite the opposite: Individuals are often drawn to the medical field out of a desire to care for others; if asked what they like most about being doctors, nurses, or therapists, they would cite the satisfactions of caring. But I submit that one can be a caring professional, endeavoring in good faith to help others, and still participate in a system that seeks to diminish and marginalize the patient. Indeed, the caring ethic masks the power inequity by convincing practitioners (and the rest of us) that because they are here to help others, no one is oppressed, no one could be victimized, and power just isn't relevant. Such is not reality, however. Politics is as real as physiology, even in the medical system.

With this in mind, then, I fashioned a set of principles that now govern my interactions with health-care professionals and the medical system and track to a great extent the manner in which I conduct my life as an individual with a disability outside of my medical needs. These standards evoke for me dozens of relevant stories, and I will share some of them by way of illustration.

First, as the person with the greatest stake in my health care, I make the decisions and no health professional can overrule my preferences. This seems, at first, a somewhat indisputable position. In practice, however, health professionals have difficulty when the decisions I make are in direct conflict with their advice or preferences. These need not even be conflicts over weighty health problems, and they quickly deteriorate into absurdity. One spring afternoon, a month or two after I had begun using a portable ventilator, I was outside getting some fresh air, strolling with one of my nurses in the park that runs down the middle of the avenue where I live. Side streets cross the park at one-block intervals, and traffic from the avenue often turns onto the side street. As I reached one of the side streets, I checked to see if cars were turning left from the avenue and approaching me from my right. Concluding that it was safe to proceed, and *not* consulting the nurse, I crossed the street.

When I reached the other side it was abundantly clear that the nurse was unhappy with what had just occurred. She stopped and said, "You should wait until I say it's safe to cross because if something happens I'm responsible." I had been living in Boston for nearly 10 years, so my first inclination was to burst out laughing, but instead I asked, "Are you responsible because I'm a fellow human being or because you're the nurse?" She replied that it was because I am a fellow human being, but neither of us believed her. I then said, "If you want to continue on this case you had better get this straight: You have no decision-making authority whatsoever. You are here for your medical advice and as an emergency backup. I am not mentally incompetent, and therefore you can't make medical decisions on my behalf, and you certainly can't decide when I cross the street. If you cannot abide by these conditions then you should not be working here." I have not seen her since. This problem is the result, at least in part, of the work experiences of nurses in intensive care units where patients are gravely ill and in need of surrogate decision makers. Some nurses cannot comprehend that home care with me is very different. But even professionals that seem to understand, that appear to "get it," will catch themselves or be caught making decisions for me and acting unilaterally. The ideology is deeply embedded.

The second principle that governs my relationship with the medical system flows from the first. As I am the only legitimate decision maker, no one else is permitted to speak for me. Again this principle seems unassailable, but in practice it is a position more often observed in the breach. Far too commonly, a doctor or nurse enters my hospital room and speaks to another professional or to a family member rather than to me. Medical staff have also tried to order for me in restaurants, make requests for me in department stores, and take it upon themselves to reprimand the concierge in my apartment building because the elevator was not working—all in the name of my health care. Such actions are not only corrosive to my self-esteem but undermine my personal interactions and professional integrity by advancing the perception that my needs are so extensive as to render me irrelevant and nearly invisible.

So if I am to speak for myself and make the decisions, it follows that I must have complete information, and that is the third principle. The system is remarkably prone to keep information about a patient's condition and treatment away from the patient, while the professionals blithely discuss patient information in crowded elevators and cafeterias. At one point in the intensive care unit I asked to see my chart. The head nurse for the unit first stated that hospital policy did not allow her to show me the chart. When I informed her that such a policy was in violation of the state patient rights law, she then said that she needed the approval of my doctor before she could produce the chart. The doctor told her that I was to have access to the chart whenever I deemed it necessary, but clearly the presumption that patients may not see their charts was well entrenched.

Another telling example was the behavior of residents during morning rounds. All of the important information and discussion about my case would occur outside of my room, before the residents came in to see me. Because my hearing is acute, I noticed that what they discussed outside was nothing like the subsequent conversation with me, so I would cut past the small talk to ask questions about the other conversation. Years of seeking complete information have transformed me into a sophisticated medical consumer, and I am no longer intimidated by medical data and technical jargon.

Failure to provide me with information about what is actually happening to me, or what the doctors do not yet know, is a cause of great frustration and even anguish. In the summer of 1992, a ventilator malfunctioned; I went into respiratory arrest and had to be resuscitated. When I regained consciousness, I was transported to the hospital and tests were undertaken to determine if there had been any neurological or cardiac damage. Early indications were that no damage had occurred, and my wife and I were told unequivocally that I would be released in 2 days. Unbeknown to the two of us, the doctors were waiting for the results of a certain enzyme test that would determine whether I could leave the hospital. On the morning I was to be released I was suddenly transferred from the intensive care unit to the cardiac care unit (CCU) with little explanation. Between the experience of nearly dying and, now, the fear elicited by this sudden and drastic change of plans, we were devastated. Add to this the aggravation of a nasty, high-handed nurse in the CCU, and the result was an incredibly stressful and upsetting situation. All this distress could have been avoided if only the doctors had told us that I could go home if the results of that last enzyme test were satisfactory.

The fourth principle of dealing with the medical system involves the role my health care is allowed to play in the rest of my life. Health care is a means to a full and meaningful life; it is not an end in itself. But because the professionals deal only with the medical aspects of my life, they often lose sight of the impact of their recommendations on my career, home life, and relationships. If their efforts are not resisted, the medical agenda will overwhelm the human agenda—the tail will wag the dog.

Consider two examples. Because the ventilator delivers air directly to the lungs, bypassing the sinuses, I am required to drink a large amount of fluid to maintain sufficient hydration. We have a system for a rough recording of the intake, and renal function has never been one of my problems. I use cups that are all larger than 240 cc (8 ounces). For convenience we record each cup as 240 cc, since the point is to take in as much fluid as possible and any excess is in our favor. One of the nurses wanted to mark all of our cups and mugs (even the wedding china!) with a china marker to indicate the exact volume contained in each. The proposal would have delighted Franz Kafka.

The second example not only reflects the attempted hegemony of the medical sphere but also illustrates how various needs must be juggled to maintain the life I desire. I have a tracheostomy, a direct opening in my throat, and am particularly susceptible to respiratory infection. Given the deterioration of my chest muscles, any infection can potentially develop into pneumonia and any pneumonia can be lethal. Some have argued, therefore, that I should eliminate all sources of risk and protect myself at all costs. But that could happen only if I were willing to live apart from other people in some kind of bubble. I would not be able to teach, represent clients, see friends, have an intimate life with my wife, play with my nephews and godchildren, or hug my dog. In other words, all those things that give my life value, purpose, and meaning would be sacrificed in order to protect me from infections that might kill me. Who would want to have such a barren, empty life? So instead we take what precautions are reasonable, in the context of the life I choose to lead, and accept the risks and the consequences of a meaningful existence. I am fully aware of the dangers, and my choices are the result of a rational decision-making process, but even if these choices are arbitrary and irrational, they are *my* choices and may not be gainsaid.

After nearly 35 years, my relationship with muscular dystrophy, like any other long-term relationship, has grown exceedingly close and complex. We have forged a bond as fellow travelers, and traveling the road together has taught me to fight but also to cherish life and the people who give that life meaning. For a long time I believed that the disease could not be real if I refused to acknowledge its existence—if I kept it out of sight. But I have always known my disease-companion to be close by, waiting just beyond my vision. Now I find that I prefer to invite my companion into the light of the fire rather than search for his eyes in the dark.

CRITICAL-THINKING ACTIVITIES

1. What are the four principles that govern attorney Macurdy's interactions with health-care professionals and the medical system? Discuss their importance for all patients and families.

2. Macurdy wants health-care professionals to understand that health care is a means to a full and meaningful life, not an end in itself. Discuss the importance of this understanding.

3. Imagine that you are a clinical instructor of medical and nursing students and it is the day in which the author's respiratory system deteriorated to the point where he needed mechanical assistance in order to breathe comfortably. How would you guide your students in inititating the iron lung, keeping in mind the four principles that this author designed? Outline your procedure in detail.

4. Explain in detail the physiological responses to terror and its effect on the body's vital organs, specifically the cardiac and respiratory systems. Discuss the reasons why it is important to take this crucial evidence into consideration when initiating the iron lung or conducting any procedure.

5. Discuss the author's evidence that certain health-care providers are locked into a "habit of mind" and a "system of beliefs" that lead them to misunderstand and to oppress.

Example c̄ nurse : her habit to be a surrogate decision-
                     maker

marginalizing   : a presumpt'n that pts may not see their
client although   charts was "well-entrenched"
masked as
caring   : a presumption that pt. doesn't need to
                     know everything

6. The author tells us that the everyday language of health-care practitioners is laden with authoritarian nuances. Compare his examples with those taken from your experience, and discuss the implications of this misuse of language.

7. Macurdy informs us that "politics is as real as physiology, even in the medical system." Discuss this phenomenon in relation to your discipline and its hierarchies, chain of command, and pattern of authority. What are the differences and similarities between the various disciplines?

8. The author reveals that at age 13 he began to learn "the social techniques to work around others' reactions to [his] disability." Discuss the importance of this learning and the ways in which you could incorporate this knowledge into your practice.

9. Compare and contrast the "habit of mind" and "system of beliefs" of the health-care professionals in this narrative with those of the author.

#9 We want to be surrogate decision makers and put ourselves in charge

We speak for pts

We fail to disclose complete info : using med jargon
charts not given to pts.

Our recommendations don't always take into consideration the 'whole' pt .

Dorothy C. Buck

Dorothy C. Buck has a PhD in religion and literature from Boston University and an MA in pastoral counseling from Emmanuel College in Boston. She also completed a 3-year certificate of postgraduate training at the Boston Institute for Psychotherapy. Dr. Buck teaches in the Graduate Program in Ministries and the Psychology Department at Emmanuel College and has a private practice as a licensed mental health practitioner in Boston. Her background includes many years as a classical ballet performer and teacher. She is the author of *The Dance of Life* (Paragon House, New York, 1987) and has published essays in *Dance Magazine*, the Carmelite journal *Living Prayer*, and *Sufi, A Journal of Sufism*.

Dr. Buck has two children, Ariane, a Stanford University graduate, and Raoul. She lives in Boston, Massachusetts, with her husband, Anselm Blumer.

When Dr. Buck's son Raoul was a toddler, his developmental delays were diagnosed as being caused by mild brain damage with some signs of cerebral palsy and mild autistic behaviors. Here she reveals the complex and simple needs and inherent struggles with teachers and health-care professionals that emerged over the last 27 years of striving to educate and help Raoul develop to his fullest potential.

CHAPTER 3

Raoul

by Dorothy C. Buck

*L*ast month we went to Connecticut to help my son Raoul move into a group home. He has been living in a state regional center for nearly 10 years. In a few weeks he will be 27 years old. When he was 2 1/2 years old, Raoul was diagnosed as a brain-damaged child with some signs of cerebral palsy and mild autistic behaviors. Like millions of babies who are born each year with brain damage, there was no apparent reason for his disability.

When I was pregnant with Raoul, I had no way of knowing that motherhood would change my life more dramatically than it would other women's lives. My husband and I were professional dancers, and I felt in exceptionally good physical condition. The pregnancy went smoothly. We hoped our baby would be born in time for our wedding anniversary. He was born at New York Hospital 2 weeks late. The year 1968 was an exciting time for the maternity unit in this hospital because "natural childbirth" was being encouraged. All the nursing staff had taken Lamaze birthing courses, and so had we. They were waiting for women like me who were ready to try it. My husband breathed with me through every contraction. Even though I know that babies are born every minute, Raoul's birth felt like a miracle to me.

In retrospect, I know that I was saved much anxiety in those early years because Raoul was my first child. I had no experience of normal infant development and didn't know enough to worry when the pediatrician suggested that Raoul's retarded motor development was due to "poor muscle tone." When Raoul was 8 months, the doctor suggested that he might have mild cerebral palsy. At 12 months he wondered if Raoul's one "weak" eye, which tended to turn inward, should be seen by a specialist in children's eye diseases. We took him to the recommended specialist. This man's interest and research were in diagnosing a particular kind of weakness in the eye muscles of infants and toddlers. He assured us that this was Raoul's problem and that cosmetic surgery would correct it at age 3.

By the time Raoul was 4 or 5 his eye had straightened out, tending to turn inward only when he was overtired. Some years later another eye doctor made far more sense when he stated that Raoul's "weak eye" was directly associated with his disability and generally slow developmental process.

Raoul began to babble, say some words, and sit up by himself. Eventually he scooted all over the apartment in a "walker." He was cute, energetic, and engaging, but was still not trying to stand on his own.

When Raoul was 14 months, our pediatrician suggested that we consult another specialist in infant diseases at New York Hospital. This doctor seemed unconcerned, suggesting that Raoul was not yet out of the normal developmental range for walking. "After all," he said, "Raoul hasn't read the textbooks on when babies are supposed to walk." We felt better.

When Raoul was 18 months old, we moved to Alabama to work with a ballet company there. Raoul could walk if you held his hands, but not yet alone. Later I discovered that friends knew there was something seriously wrong, but no one discussed it with us. The pediatrician in Alabama had Raoul's eyes tested, then his hearing, which he thought might be responsible for the slow development. What about his very flexible joints? Raoul could sit for long periods of time, even fall asleep, with his knees flopped open to the floor and his body slumped forward. His hip-joint x rays were normal. When we returned to New York a year later, I found out that there was a very progressive research center for child development in Alabama. No one had suggested it. Raoul was 2 1/2 and still not walking on his own.

We took Raoul back to New York Hospital to the same specialist in early infant diseases who had seen him at 14 months. This time he suggested a full neurological evaluation. Raoul's electroencephalogram read normal. His speech evaluation suggested that he was on the low side of normal development. Finally, a team of doctors at the Cerebral Palsy Clinic evaluated his motor development. His fine motor skills were within normal range. Although Raoul crawled with the appropriate opposition of knees and arms, he was fearful of moving from sitting to lying down backward. His motor skills appeared to be developing normally, but the process was markedly slow. The occupational therapist suggested getting Raoul a small chair that he could push in front of him to help him walk. At that time the diagnosis was mild brain damage with some indication of mild cerebral palsy. I was not yet able to imagine what this would mean for our family as Raoul grew up.

We were now living in Connecticut, where we found a wonderful pediatrician. I'll never forget that first meeting. He asked us to come at 5 PM after office hours so that we would have more time. As I was filling Dr. W. in on our son's history he showed Raoul a cabinet filled with toys. After emptying the cabinet Raoul found an appropriate-size chair and took off down the hall to explore. Dr. W. observed Raoul's behavior, got down on the floor with him to play, and finally suggested that Raoul had many interesting qualities that did not entirely fit with the diagnosis from New York Hospital. He was bright-eyed and engaging, for one, and he had no fear of leaving me to go exploring out of my sight by himself. He wondered what the Yale Child Study Center would say.

Once someone said to me that "special" children are gifts from God given to families who know how to love and care for them. It has always felt to me that I learned how to care for Raoul because I had to in order to meet the needs of those I love. I have no question that Raoul is a gift to everyone he meets. One time we were visiting a friend who lived in a religious community. An older man was cutting the lawn while sitting on the seat of an electric mower, which fascinated Raoul. My friend cautioned us that this man was not very friendly. Raoul took off toward the noisy mower and suddenly the noise stopped. We watched in amazement while Raoul happily talked the man into taking him for a ride on the mower.

I am able to see only in retrospect that the gift to me was the challenge to my own growth as a person and to become the mother that Raoul needed. For many years I felt exhausted and often burdened by the many battles for Raoul's well-being that lay ahead.

As an infant and toddler, Raoul didn't seem to require more attention except that he was probably in a stroller longer than most. In those years I only partially heard the pediatrician's concern. I called my obstetrician to verify a normal birth process, took

Raoul to specialists, and tried to drown out the gnawing thoughts that I was somehow responsible for Raoul's disability. Should I have continued dancing and teaching into my ninth month? When he had an ear infection and high fever at age 3 months and we were told to give him a cold bath and enema to lower his temperature, did it damage his brain?

One day while I was teaching in the studio, I left Raoul in the large waiting area with a baby-sitter. At a break I came out and she said, "You know, Raoul is walking!" He came into the studio with me and for the next hour and a half exuberantly crawled to a wall, climbed to his feet, and walked all around the room until he fell down. He repeated the exercise over and over. He was excited, and so was I. Raoul was now 3 1/2 years old.

It took several more years for Raoul to feel confident enough to step down from a curb to the street. Instead, he would sit on the curb and climb down. It took even more years for him to walk down steps without needing to place both feet securely on each step, one at a time. He continues to hold onto railings with both hands and is more fearful of escalators now than he was as a little child. It is my experience that physical development and coordination are directly related to mental ability and alertness. My intuition as a dancer suggested that I could help my son developmentally by seeking out some kind of rehabilitation program. I took Raoul to the Rehabilitation Center. This was the beginning of my many frustrated creative efforts to help Raoul. I was told that these programs were not suitable for him because his disability was developmental rather than the result of physical injury. If I had had the financial resources I might have been able to find a gym with someone willing to work with my child. Nautilus did not exist at the time, but it might have been a perfect solution. Late walking, along with Raoul's tendency to favor one side, resulted in some severe problems that might have been avoided if I had been successful in finding a strengthening and stabilizing physical rehabilitation program when he began to walk.

Beyond the physical advantages, it is clear to me that the emotional effects of feeling strong, especially if the undeveloped side of Raoul's body were strengthened, would surely provide a sense of physical security and an accompanying emotional assurance. Certainly, the tentative aspects of Raoul's personality are partially due to experiencing a physical world that is unstable and awkward. Instead, Raoul's calf muscles remained underdeveloped, and over time one foot became deformed, as it was increasingly used less than the other. By the time he was 12, the effect on Raoul's lower back was sufficient to be diagnosed as scoliosis. Surgery was advised for his lame foot. By lengthening his Achilles tendon and subsequently having him wear a brace for the remainder of his growing years, we managed to avoid the worst effects of scoliosis. He is left with one foot two sizes smaller than the other. Shoes are an ongoing problem.

Raoul is a survivor in the most meaningful sense of the word. The Children's Hospital accommodated our "special needs" by putting a cot for me by Raoul's bed so that I could be with him through the night before and after surgery. He did very well. By the second day he was in a wheelchair, his leg propped up in a cast, asking me to push him all over the hospital. When friends came to visit, we went out onto the grounds. Before long, Raoul was pushing the wheels himself, and laughing uproariously while my friend pushed him up a high ramp and raced down it with him at high speed. Raoul had his very own roller coaster, and loved it.

Once Raoul began to walk, his slow development and limited ability to do things for himself began to become irritating and frustrating to me, a person who easily juggled three activities at once and tended to think and move like a dancer, quickly and efficiently. As Raoul grew older, it seemed that the challenge to my patience increased. His developing vocabulary was the most confusing and difficult. He was learning by imitation, but it was not clear that the words had any meaning for him. Along with this is what psychologists today might describe as attention deficit disorder. We called it extreme distractibility. It seemed that Raoul heard every sound in his immediate environment. The telephone ringing in another apartment, a truck going by outside, or a horn blowing. Words from the conversation of people sitting at a table behind us in a restaurant would be interjected into Raoul's chatter. His speech was clear, but made little sense. This stage was the most painful because I never knew for sure what Raoul understood. I have vivid memories of getting angry at him for breaking something or for stuffing the toilet with toilet paper so that it overflowed, and realizing that when I asked if he knew what he had done, all he knew was that I was angry. How could I teach him not to touch a hot stove, not to turn on scalding water, if he had no way to conceptualize what he was doing or memory of what he had done? At 6 and 8 and 10, he was still very much like a 2-year-old. Every time I felt angry I also felt guilty and helpless.

One day Raoul wanted to go outside in the courtyard to play. It was late fall and cold, so I said, "Yes, you can go out, but first put on your jacket." As I went to get the jacket Raoul started screaming that he wanted to go outside. Nothing helped to calm him down until I got him outside with his jacket on.

I took him to the Yale Child Study Center hoping to find someone to help me discern what Raoul understood and to encourage more appropriate speech. One young woman was willing to try but moved elsewhere after a few months. No one else took an interest; I later learned that developmental studies are focused on "normal" children. It appears we are not able to learn anything significant about developmental processes from brain-damaged or mentally retarded children. But I did, because every stage of learning new skills took so much longer for Raoul that each tiny step in the process was magnified and clear.

When Raoul was still an infant he began to make a humming noise while he ate. As he got older the humming seemed to be associated with his concentration. Perhaps it was a way to block out internal and external interference. The humming became a kind of droning. Even though it was annoying, it had an advantage because it allowed me to be able to let Raoul play outside in the yard. I could always hear where he was. Despite his physical limitations, Raoul maintained his curiosity and urge to explore. This resulted in many instances of losing him in the mall or when he was playing outside in the neighborhood. The local police came to know him well; this only added to my increasing anxiety.

When Raoul was 3 1/2, I gave birth to a little girl. The story that best exemplifies her early experience of her brother also identifies another source of my own anxiety. They were about 3 and 6 years old and sitting on the kitchen floor with ice cream cones. In an aggressive 3-year-old moment she grabbed Raoul's cone out of his hand. To her amazement he did nothing. He just sat and watched her with tears in his eyes. From then on, she states, she knew that in some way she would need to protect her older brother.

One of the many stories that I have come to call "Raoul's lost stories" happened about the same time on a very hot day when we decided to go to the beach. At that time Raoul was carrying a little notebook and pencil around with him. He liked to ask people to write for him while he dictated what they should say. It was a holiday and the beach was very crowded. The campgrounds surrounding the beach area were full of camper trailers and people enjoying cookouts. As we made our way from the car to the beach, Raoul's sister had to go to the bathroom. I left Raoul with his father standing on the crowded boardwalk. When we returned, I didn't see him. "He was right here a minute ago," exclaimed his father. We gave the lifeguards a description of our curly blond-haired child with great blue eyes and long eyelashes, and for the remainder of the day we scoured the beach. I knew that Raoul was afraid of the water and was not likely to go near the waves by himself. Nevertheless, the more time that went by, the more frightened I became.

After 3 in the afternoon the beach began to clear, and by late afternoon we could scan the length of it. By then we had contacted the security police. They suggested my husband accompany them on their rounds of the campgrounds. Within the hour they returned with my son, happily clutching his notebook, his mouth covered with ketchup. There was a message written on his notepad. "I enjoyed meeting you, Raoul. I hope you liked the hot dog." It was signed Nancy. The time was 7 PM. Apparently Raoul had followed some folks into the campgrounds, and everyone assumed he belonged to someone there. Although I call these stories "Raoul's lost stories," he himself is never lost. He knows where he is and assumes we do too. As he wandered from one campsite to another, probably talking to people who would talk to him, I imagine he asked in his usual way, "What are you doing?" which was Raoul's way of saying, "Can I have one too?" Apparently "Nancy" understood Raoul's language.

Raoul's unguarded innocence is his special gift, but like many of his qualities, it occasionally puts him in danger. To this day Raoul is sure that he knows everyone, that no one is a stranger. He walks up to people in the grocery store and says, "I like that bag. What's in it?" or "I know you, what's your name?" One time he went down another aisle while I was looking for something. When I found him, he was face to face with a man who was obviously drunk and angry. "If you bother me one more time, kid—" the man was saying. Without thinking I put myself between them explaining that Raoul was disabled and meant no harm. I was lucky. The man went off grumbling something to himself.

Sometimes Raoul was taken advantage of by other children in the neighborhood, but fortunately there were older children who came to take him out to play and were very kind to him. I heard many stories from other parents who were not so lucky.

Every new skill was an exciting breakthrough for Raoul. When he was 5 he learned to ride a tricycle for the first time, and by 8 he rode a bicycle with training wheels. But when he outgrew small bicycles, there were no training wheels made for bikes his size. I still feel sad every time Raoul asks for a 10-speed bike or talks about riding one.

When Raoul was 3 1/2 I was introduced to the world of special education. For 2 years the nursery school for "special" children provided me with some help for a few hours a day in teaching Raoul some important functional skills and offered a social environment for Raoul. He entered kindergarten and moved through the classrooms of a school for mentally retarded children. He was classified as trainable mentally retarded (TMR). From then on the battles with the school board began as Raoul's limitations became increasingly evident.

It seems to me that classrooms for TMR children are designed to appease the fears of both educators and parents. Efforts at "normalization" avoid the pain and reality of differences. Those children who are mildly retarded may have the potential to learn to read or write and recognize numbers. Telling time and naming the months of the year are often within their range of ability. Therefore, the classroom is designed to function as much like normal school as possible. It became increasingly evident, however, that all of these children are unique in their disabilities and, therefore, their different potentials. Children like Raoul very quickly begin to fall through the cracks in the system. By the time Raoul was 8 it was very clear to me that Raoul was going to have to learn the functional skills necessary to live in the world without knowing how to read, write, or recognize numbers.

At home we struggled to teach Raoul how to button buttons, zip zippers, put on socks and shoes, wash his hands, and brush his teeth. Every morning I tried to make sure he went to the bathroom just minutes before the bus came, often with no success. Even though he wore rubber pants and plastic diapers, Raoul seemed to purposely wait to soil everything he had on until the moment the bus appeared. I became a master at quick changes while the bus driver patiently waited for Raoul. He was finally relatively toilet-trained by age 10, although even now he may wet his bed in a new environment. I learned to carry a change of clothing and a roll of toilet paper everywhere we went.

Meanwhile Raoul's sister seemed to me to be on developmental fast-forward. Raoul had played happily in a playpen for years. She had no tolerance for it. By 13 months she was running around, and by 3 she was toilet-trained, tying shoelaces, and attempting to imitate the dancers in my advanced ballet classes. It was a revelation for me. She soon had friends and playmates, and another painful issue arose. I asked Raoul's teachers if there was another child like him so that I could find him a playmate too. I went to PTA meetings hoping to meet another mother with a similar request. I had no luck. Apparently no other child in this school was quite like Raoul or in need of a playmate.

The principal of Raoul's school agreed with me that the programs were not designed to meet Raoul's specific needs. I learned the words "functional daily living skills." Such programs existed for nonverbal children. Raoul's verbal ability disqualified him. While Raoul became stronger and more resistant to my efforts to help him learn to shower and dress himself, I battled with school boards in an effort to find a program to meet Raoul's needs. I was informed that it was my job to teach him daily living skills and the school's job to teach him "academics." This is an altogether unreasonable demand. Children need clear role distinctions and a nurturing mother figure at home to act as a buffer against the inevitable frustrations at school. Of course, mothers teach their children many things in everyday living, but I believe that children need Mom to be Mom so that their teachers can be teachers.

The board of education suggested a new community regional school. Raoul was placed in a classroom with autistic children, most of whom were nonverbal and learning to use sign language. Many were more capable academically and functionally than Raoul. The philosophy in this school was to sign to every child while simultaneously speaking the words. Raoul started waving his hands around and began to lose eye contact when he was talking. I was told that "experts" agreed that signing was good for Raoul because it "reinforced" his language, but no one actually taught him the signs. My research informed me that once a child learns to speak a word, the sign should be discontinued to "reinforce" speaking. I was outraged. It took 2 years to find a more suitable school on my own and convince the board of education to provide transportation for Raoul to another district.

My feeling in these planning meetings was that I was not being heard or given credibility for my knowledge and experience with my own son. Although it was a legal option for parents to be involved, I experienced a division between me and the "professionals" that created a discouraging tension. Parents were perceived as untrained, uneducated, and lacking in expertise. Yet, I knew his strengths and limitations better than anyone. I had the real story in relation to Raoul's needs.

The school I found had a very active gym program and a teacher who recognized that physical exercise was a valuable developmental tool. Raoul was programmed for gym every day, and along with walking up and down steps and bicycling, he learned to jump on a trampoline.

Raoul's unique abilities have puzzled psychologists for years and left me searching for the mysterious key that might open the door to learning for my son. I repeatedly tried to encourage his teachers to take advantage of his interests and strengths as a means of motivating him to learn boring things like letters and numbers. I had little doubt that he would never learn to read or write, but I was struck by his amazing ability to distinguish between a telephone company van and a police van. He always knows the ice cream truck and points out all the Honda Civics or cars that look like those owned by our friends. If you ask Raoul to name the color of something, he will name a color, although it may not be the right one. The same is true of girls' names, or street names, or highway route numbers. He has an uncanny ability to categorize and recognize the things in his environment, like the names of supermarkets and gasoline stations, which we assume require an ability to read.

It seemed to me that Raoul's desire to be helpful could be a tool for boosting his self-esteem while teaching him useful functional skills like counting. Sorting the silverware, putting it in the appropriate space in a drawer, and setting the table seemed a far more appropriate way to teach Raoul to count, sort, and categorize than having him work with colored disks or flash cards. The common rewards of colored stars or candy for completing a task failed miserably with Raoul and reveal a misuse of the behavioral methods commonly used in our schools. Raoul needed teachers who were eager to find creative ways to engage him and tap into his own motivation to learn. Instead, his experience was boredom, failure, and an increasing lack of self-confidence. In spite of all this, Raoul found ingenious ways of coping with his insufficiencies. He learned to change the subject if he was asked anything that he didn't know. While observing some psychological testing through a two-way mirror, I watched Raoul lose interest, yawn incessantly, and ask irrelevant questions throughout the session. Yet, sit Raoul at a musical keyboard with its many wonderful sounds and rhythms and he will be absorbed for hours, easily learning to plug it in and turn the power on himself. He has mastered radios, Walkman tape recorders, and television sets and even managed to find the invisible compartment on my computer and turn the light off for the screen when I was busy in another room. I was sure that something was wrong with the computer until I finally found the hidden buttons.

The new school programmed Raoul for speech therapy a few times a week. The goal was appropriate responses, and Raoul began to learn how to say "I don't know" rather than change the subject, and how to ask for information.

Raoul grew up in my ballet studio. Music was as much a part of his world as it was mine. When he was about 4 he was sitting watching class by the piano in the studio while I walked around clapping or counting out the rhythm for the dancers. At one moment I stopped and was stunned to hear the sound of clapping behind me as Raoul gleefully continued to keep perfect rhythm with the music.

We all liked to sing together, especially Christmas carols. Raoul knew a lot of the words but often preferred to make up his own while we joined in, following his lead and laughing hysterically: "We wish you a merry Christmas, Raoul's here with Mom for Christmas, Raoul's here with Mom for Christmas, the keys to the car."

When Raoul was 8 years old I became a single parent. The stress of parenting was compounded by financial constraints and the logistics of caretaking without a partner. The stress took its toll on my physical health as well. I was forced to learn about our social system the hard way. Although I was connected to a social worker through Raoul's school, I was not informed of the social services available to us until Raoul was 10 years old. His disability made him eligible for Social Security Supplemental Income (SSI), a small but very helpful addition to my unreliable income. Baby-sitters became harder to find as Raoul got older and harder to manage. I discovered we could apply for respite care through the state Department of Mental Retardation (DMR). Raoul spent an occasional weekend at a state regional center or with a respite-care family. Thus we began a long relationship with the Connecticut DMR, which continues to this day.

As I struggled to support my small family, I came face to face with my own need for support both emotionally and spiritually. When I got in touch with Association for Retarded Citizens (ARC), an active group of parents with special-needs children, I encountered the frightening legal and political realities that would directly affect Raoul's education and future life. The tension and anxiety that I saw on the faces of these other parents reinforced my own fears and became intolerable. At that time I had to concentrate on providing the best I could for Raoul and his sister. I didn't have the energy for political lobbying for more years of education or services, despite their obvious importance.

I relied on my friends, many of whom had known Raoul since he was 2 1/2, and found a supporting church community. Raoul attended a preparatory class for First Communion and Confirmation designed for special-needs children. I developed an ever-deepening prayer life that was sustained by weekend retreats with a community of religious sisters who provided friendship and love, a container for my anxiety, and nourishment for my aching heart. My fears for Raoul's future were not unfounded, and my sorrow that he would never have so many of life's experiences remains as a kind of chronic grief hidden somewhere deep within me.

Taking Raoul to church was an experience for everyone. He soon learned the Lord's Prayer and joined in for much of the singing. It became disconcerting for some, however, when Raoul's voice could be heard repeating the words of the priest at the opening of the Liturgy. "In the name of the Father, and the Son, and the Holy Spirit," the priest proclaimed. "In the name of the Father, and the Son, and the Holy Spirit," echoed Raoul in a loud voice. One of my cherished memories is the look of pleasure on Raoul's face when I solved the problem of my being interrupted by letting him say grace for us: "Thank you, Lord, for this food, amen," followed by Raoul's contagious laughter.

Many years ago a friend of mine took my children and hers to a beach at the bottom of a rocky slope. Later she told me that she sat with Raoul on the rocks watching the other children race down the slope to the sandy beach below. Suddenly she heard Raoul's barely audible voice mutter, "Maybe someday I can do that." Truly a lucid moment, for even today Raoul is more likely to say something like, "I did that yesterday." We all know what he means, but we can only imagine what he might have been feeling.

The precariousness of Raoul's physical life was evident in the many accidents that had us racing him to the emergency room for stitches. He fell on coffee tables, hit his head on the bathroom sink, and had his front baby teeth sewn back in at the age of 4. Today, however, his awkwardness is a distinct aspect of his charm. There is no more endearing moment than when Raoul throws his arms around a friend for a totally spontaneous hug. And my heart is always touched when we are driving in the car and out of the blue Raoul says, "I like you, Mom."

When Raoul's permanent teeth came in it was clear that he had an overbite that should be corrected. The orthodontist was adamant that the overbite was caused by Raoul's thumb sucking and until that ceased there was nothing to be done. "Years ago, they removed molars and put in permanent braces, but that is not done anymore. In fact," he explained, "we expect children to be able to participate in their treatment today by using retainers that they must wear at certain times. Do you think Raoul would be capable of doing that?" I didn't know if Raoul's thumb sucking was a cause or not, but I did know that my own brother had 5 years of permanent braces as a child. Heredity seemed like a more reasonable explanation.

At the time I had the sense that there was another issue at stake here—that it was very important for Raoul to look as "normal" as possible. I knew that correcting Raoul's teeth would affect the shape of his face and jawline. As a little child he was beautiful to look at, with his blond curls and long dark eyelashes highlighting his big blue eyes. Surely the fact that he was so cute was part of his "acceptability" to teachers and friends. I feared his rejection by a not-so-kind world if he also looked too different. And worst of all, I wasn't sure if the orthodontist was really suggesting that a child like Raoul was not worth the effort. Perhaps I was overreacting.

Raoul's anxiety was often hard to predict or understand. He loved going to school on the bus, but he had no tolerance for waiting. I will never forget the tension we felt every morning getting Raoul dressed for school. I purposely attempted to quietly encourage him to help me get him ready, hoping to keep him calm. One particular morning a friend called just as Raoul's frustration with a sleeve that was turned inside out reached its peak. "I don't want to go to school. I hate the bus!" screamed Raoul, as he flung his shoe across the room. "Do you need help?" asked my concerned friend. I explained that these outbursts were common on some mornings. What made him anxious one day and not the next was a mystery. I couldn't help feeling responsible and wondered if he was sensitive to the time pressure that I felt, or worried that the bus wouldn't come, or acting out his own frustration with dressing skills.

When Raoul was 13 I picked him up from an after-school program at the regional center. He was upset because we couldn't find his hat. I told him we had another one at home. He continued to ask about his hat as we drove home, and no amount of reassurance calmed his increasing agitation. As we climbed the steps to our apartment he began to escalate into a tantrum, screaming and crying, arms flailing in every direction. When we entered the apartment I told him to go into his room until he could calm down. He did as he was told, and the next thing I heard was the sound of glass breaking. When I rushed into the room, Raoul was sitting on the bed, stunned into silence. He had smashed the window with his fist. Raoul was not hurt, but I became abruptly aware of my limitations and the danger of injury and accidents that were real possibilities. Raoul was becoming too big for me to control, and I would not always be able to protect him or those around him. I had visions of having to call the police for help.

In my efforts to find a safer living environment for Raoul I researched boarding schools all over New England to no avail. The board of education would never pay for it. Finally a friend offered to take Raoul as her first client in a community training home (CTH). The state had created a program of foster care as alternative living arrangements for DMR clients. We tried it. After 2 years Raoul was returned to me for no clear reason. The social workers assured me they were trying to find another CTH, but the 3-month time limit elapsed and he was taken off the client list. Now I was in a battle with the state. I went from social workers to supervisors to the superintendent of the regional center. I was told that there were no placements in the entire state. Finally one was found, but it meant that Raoul also had to change schools. I was caught in a terrible dilemma. Raoul's school placement was very important, but if I didn't take this opportunity to get him back into the state system we might not get another chance. I had to compromise. The placement lasted 3 months when I discovered that the provider was abusing his clients. They were removed from his home. My worst nightmares were being realized. I had fantasies of being 95 years old and desperately trying to stay alive to take care of my son.

Raoul was placed in another home. Within a year this woman found Raoul's need for help with daily living skills, and inability to be left alone in a room without taking the TV apart, too demanding. We put our heads together and I called the state commissioner for the DMR. Within days Raoul was evaluated by the state psychologist, and a recommendation for placement was agreed upon. Raoul moved to a year-old state regional center on Holy Thursday of Easter week in 1985. At the time he needed the structure and the safety of an institutional environment. Raoul was finally in a setting where functional daily living skills were programmed into his overall plan of care. He was 17 years old.

When Raoul moved into the center, one of his most endearing qualities emerged. Almost immediately he befriended a woman who was not ambulatory. From then on he took his new friend out for walks in her wheelchair, often visited the women's unit after school, and was invited to join them for dinner. When I came to see him, he asked to go shopping. "Can I buy her some earrings?" he would ask. "She likes them."

Raoul's caretaking instincts were encouraged inadvertently by the fact that few of his housemates were verbal, and those that were spoke less intelligibly than Raoul. In the 10 years that he lived on campus, Raoul inevitably sought out the staff to satisfy his need to talk, sometimes incessantly, as a way of connecting to people and gratifying his need for attention. He began to identify with staff. He knew everything that was going on, who was out sick this week, who was covering, and who would be there when he returned from a day off campus with me. In the end it was decided that he needed to be included in the staff meetings rather than told not to bother people. It worked well, and by the time he was ready to move to a group home he had learned to answer the phone and get the appropriate person. I was told by the recreation director that he was an enormous help on trips to the YMCA for swimming and bowling outings. He always made sure that everyone else was in the pool or set up for bowling before he joined the activity himself. One time they even mistook him for staff at the YMCA and counted his hours for a paycheck!

There were many rewards of going to school and living in a small Connecticut town. When the age level of the special classes that Raoul attended outgrew the grammar school, his teacher worked hard to convince the local high school to give these special-needs students classroom space. There were the doubts and heightened anxieties of teachers and some out-and-out prejudices to overcome, but she succeeded and enhanced the experience of many of the students in the school. When Raoul graduated with his special class from high school, he was known by many of the graduating seniors. I'll never forget the graduation ceremony. It happened to be the high school's 100th anniversary. There was Raoul, dressed up in a maroon and white cap and gown, marching in with the cheering graduating class. He was the last student to be called up to the stage for his diploma. Someone helped him up the steps, and he ambled across the stage in his awkward way, laughing and waving as the crowded auditorium applauded his achievement. I cried. His certificate, which looks just like a regular high school graduation diploma, states that he attended high school. In the midst of their excitement and picture taking many students warmly called out to Raoul by name and congratulated him.

Over the years I became increasingly sensitive to Raoul's need for stability in his world, and that included trying to bring people into his life who would not disappear. It was confusing for Raoul to learn a new friend's name, which sometimes took several visits, and then not see that person again. He was likely to call the next person I brought by the previous person's name and "forget," or not be able to absorb, the new information. In 1991, I remarried. My marriage created a new stability as we continued to visit regularly and bring Raoul home several times a year. He became attached to my husband and often asks to speak to him when I call. Our home visits, for holidays or his birthday, require several days when we can give him our undivided attention. We take him on buses and subways all over the city, or on anything that moves, as my daughter says. We invite many friends for gatherings where Raoul can be included. He adds his presence to the conversations by interrupting with questions or statements that some-times make no sense and other times are shockingly accurate. The keyboard is set up on a stand in the living room with headphones so that Raoul can play when he gets bored and still be in the midst of the party. He indiscriminately pushes keys that create rhythms and inevitably arrives at the demo over and over again. Sometimes he sings along or yells out, "Listen to that, Mom!" sure that I can also hear what he is listening to with his earphones on.

Although Raoul's younger sister has now graduated from college, she continues to love and care for her brother. On her many adventures traveling around the world she faithfully sends him cards and calls often from her home in California. Raoul always tells me when she has called, although it is unclear whether it was this week or last, yes-terday or 3 days ago. "My sister called," he says. "Great!" I answer. "What did she say?" "She's coming to see me. . . . Mom, am I going to a wedding or something?" I was delighted that Raoul's godmother's son invited him to his wedding in New York City. Our children grew up together, and therefore Raoul was to be included.

It is always a challenge to take Raoul to public events. We never know for sure how he will respond, but we can be relatively sure that he won't just sit quietly. In this case, because he was part of the extended family, he sat in the second row and I silently crossed my fingers. As the wedding party proceeded down the aisle, Raoul beckoned them to "move faster" and then sat attentively until the very end of the ceremony. In the hushed silence when the groom kissed his new bride, Raoul's voice was heard from the midst of the seated guests, "Oh, how good!" he stated emphatically. Many people felt that Raoul had innocently stated the feelings of everyone there for them.

For every positive experience there is also a painful counterpart. With staff changes and insecurity in the state system, Raoul went through a difficult and unhappy period. We have been led to believe that our emotional life, and in fact our very souls as human beings, are dependent upon our memory, will, and reason. Spiritual life has been rele-gated to our superior mental capacities and the unique nature of the human mind. If we could not imagine existential issues, we are told, then, like animals, we would not have souls. Likewise, if we cannot recognize our feelings and name them, then we must have a limited emotional experience. There is no question that Raoul expresses his will, and reasonings, in his own way. His memory is also peculiarly his own. Does he truly not remember the staff person who leaves or the client who dies? Or has he learned through the many disappointments and changes in his world to block painful feelings just like you and I?

My weekly telephone calls often found him being punished for screaming inap-propriate language or telling me, "Tom doesn't like me." When I tried to find out what was happening, he would sometimes start to cry. The staff reassured me that the changes were getting to everyone, including Raoul. When I took him out for a day, he would comment strangely on the neighborhood we were driving in. "This is a nice neighborhood," he would say. "It's very quiet." Shortly before returning him to the cen-ter he would become very quiet and ask, "Why do I have to go back?" I would leave him standing at the window of his bedroom watching me wave as I drove away. He was clearly upset, and I was feeling tortured. More and more clients were being placed on his unit who had major behavioral issues and therefore required more of the staff's attention. The noise level increased. Raoul had a hard time finding a way to get atten-tion and sometimes mimicked the behaviors around him to do so. It was time to find a suitable group home.

Raoul entered a community vocational-training program. This program was estab-lished by a private agency that not only trains mentally disabled people to do routine piece work for local factories but also tries to place as many people as possible in appropriate work settings in the community. Raoul has worked in the state parks in the spring and summer on a work crew, cleaning the campsites or painting and scraping the barrels that are used by highway construction crews. He has done yard work and house-cleaning, some jobs more successfully than others. His inclination is to talk more than work and his short attention span poses problems, but he is supervised, sometimes one to one, and earns wages according to his work output. He works every day for nearly 6 hours and talks a lot about being taken for pizza by his supervisor. Best of all, Raoul gets a paycheck just like the rest of us and is learning to spend his own money for things he wants. It has been difficult for Raoul to understand that he has to give his money away in order to get a tape or a watch in return. His own money, even just a dollar or two, is very important to him.

This is his town and everywhere we go we meet someone who knows Raoul. In Caldor we meet staff from other units, at the movies we run into someone who once worked at the high school, and at the state fairs in the fall we inevitably encounter a group from one of the group homes in Raoul's town. Despite the advantages of a small town, one piece has been consistently unavailable to him. None of his peers at the center have ever been as verbal as Raoul. His verbal ability and idiosyncratic low functioning level leave him in a kind of no-man's-land. His many warm relationships have been with the staff on his unit. Our search for an appropriate group home was focused on this dilemma. We were still looking for a pal for Raoul.

It took 2 years to find a suitable placement for Raoul. We held our usual quarterly and annual team meetings, called OPS (overall plan of service), and continued to outline Raoul's needs. We felt strongly that he should be placed in the same general area so that he could keep his work program and familiar environment. We hoped to find a home with four to six clients, some of whom would be verbal like Raoul. Limiting the location also limited the possibilities. At the same time, state cutbacks and the poor economy meant no new homes were being established. The few openings that came up were often taken by clients with more pressing circumstances than Raoul. Every few months I contacted the social worker and tried to discern if I needed to also call the DMR state officials myself, as I had to do when Raoul was originally placed at the center.

At last we found Raoul's new home and began the meetings necessary to make a good transition. We talked about encouraging the staff at the center to continue to stay connected to him. His sister came to one of these meetings on one of her trips home and visited the new house with me. No one wanted this move to fail, or for Raoul to become upset and disoriented. Our fears were realistic, but Raoul fooled all of us. He has easily absorbed himself into his new life with two other verbal roommates in a mixed-gender home. He is making new friends with the staff and continuing his connections with staff and clients in his work program.

For many years Raoul has been intrigued with buying small address books in which we write my address and phone number along with his sister's, godmother's, and one of his sister's friends whom he is attached to. We added those of the staff at the center who were closest to Raoul as well. The staff at his new home soon realized that Raoul likes to call people. In the first few weeks I was hearing from friends in Rhode Island and his godmother in Syracuse that Raoul had called them. "What if I want to call my sister?" asked Raoul. "Will they dial for me?" "How did you call me here?" he wanted to know when I first began calling him at his new home.

As Raoul has grown into a young man, his speech has become more appropriate. He has a delightful sense of humor and is very affectionate and caring. He continues to seem "spacey" for brief moments from time to time. Some years ago, when he was still in school, the occupational therapist was concerned that these moments indicated mild seizure activity, but that was never clearly verified. When he gets excited he squeezes his hands together near his face, and still bites his sleeves and his knuckles. When he is tired, or feels affectionate, he continues to suck his thumb and has to be reminded to stop. He has a very limited sense of time. He knows the words for "today," "yesterday," "tomorrow," or "last week," but uses them indiscriminately. Raoul lives in the "now" of his immediate experience. He is always where he is because he has no ability to imagine being anywhere else. When he talks about memories of taking the bus to Harvard Square when he was visiting in Boston, he speaks in the present tense. I have envied Raoul's clear spiritual presence to the now of his experience. When I can be where he is with him, I enter Raoul's world, and by necessity am relieved for a while from the complexity of my own life.

I sometimes come home to messages on my machine that are unmistakable. A long silence with some noise in the background and then his voice, "Ah, what shall I say?" fading as he hangs up the receiver. A conversation with Raoul is an experience. When I call him, he often says, "Lucky, I called you." "Yes, it is," I agree. "Mom!" "Yes, Raoul." "Mom, listen to me." "I'm listening." "Say it again, I can't hear you. . . . Can I tell you something?" "Sure." "Lucky I got this money from work. My sister called me." "She did?" "What are you doing Thursday?" "Thursday I'm working, but I'm coming to see you Saturday." "You are? Tell me, wait, let me get staff." "Wait, Raoul, don't leave, they already know!" "Mom?" "Yes, Raoul." "I like you. Bye." As he goes to put the phone on the hook I hear a loud, "Yes!"

Does Raoul know that he is missing out on so much of life's experience? Is he aware of his difference? Sometimes I think so, but I'll probably never know for sure. Raoul remains innocent and is therefore one of the more vulnerable members of our society. I continue to worry about him. How will he cope with life when I am no longer here for him? But then I remember how many people have already been touched by Raoul, like the man on the power mower, and the staff at the center who love him, and now the staff in his new group home and his new roommates.

In the Special Olympics this year Raoul fast-walked 400 meters and seemed to come in fourth. I was surprised when they called him for a gold medal until we realized that he was first because he was the only one competing in his age group! But he legitimately won the gold for his softball throw. I remember the years of trying to teach him to throw a ball at all and marvel at his accomplishments. I'm left with some of my own dearest memories, like putting Raoul to bed, closing the door, and hearing "Mom?" "Yes, Raoul." "What if the bus doesn't come?" "Don't worry, it will come in the morning. Go to sleep." "Mom?" "Don't worry, I love you."

CRITICAL-THINKING ACTIVITIES

1. In your opinion, did Raoul's parents receive adequate guidance regarding growth and development of their son? What would you suggest as guiding principles for such important work?

2. What are the physical and behavioral manifestations noted by the author that would or would not support the premise that Raoul had brain damage? Cerebral palsy? Mild autistic behavior? Elaborate.

3. Do you imagine that Raoul's parents might have blamed themselves for his developmental problems? Discuss, noting evidence from this account. How might you have assisted them?

4. Dr. Buck suggests that Raoul's sense of sureness and integrity is affected negatively by his weakened right side. Do you think this is a valid premise? How do you explain this phenomenon? Discuss fully.

5. How does Raoul's distractibility affect his behavior? His relationships with others? How could he be assisted in counteracting this reality?

6. Give examples from this account of Raoul's perception of others in his life. Is he aware of dangerous situations or people? How would he communicate his awareness? Elaborate.

7. How does Raoul demonstrate his sense of others in terms of his attachments to them? Give examples from the account.

8. Is Raoul sensitive? How has he shown his capacity for understanding loss, sorrow, joy, or relief?

9. Is Raoul capable of thinking critically? What type of thinking is Raoul displaying when he assumes that others know where he is when he wanders away from his parents or thinks he called them when in reality they made the call? Discuss fully.

10. Explain the reasons why it is crucial in the diagnostic, assessment, and evaluative stage of clinical work to encourage the parents to tell narratives and stories about the child and the family. Explain how this would help to provide realistic data on what is working, what isn't, and where something different should be considered. Give examples of the possibilites of such work with narratives revealed in this account. Take into consideration what this modality could accomplish for the parents.

11. Why is it essential for educational and health-care professionals to understand the day-to-day difficulties that are a reality for Raoul and his parents? How could not knowing, and not wishing to know, create unnecessary difficulties for his family? Elaborate.

12. What factors led to Raoul's "falling through the cracks" of so many educational and rehabilitation programs? Discuss, incorporating details from the author's account. Do you think the failures of such programs has to do with the habits of mind or systems of belief held by certain administrators and other professionals? Use the explanation for "habit of mind" and "systems of belief" outlined by Macurdy in Chapter 2, "Mastery of Life."

Gertrude Simpson

Gertrude Simpson is an 11-year-old sixth grader who enjoys playing the piano and composing music. She is involved in community theater both as an actress and in set building.

Gertrude was born 8 weeks prematurely with multiple systems abnormality. Her parents were told that babies born with MSA never survive beyond the first year without surgical correction, that she would never learn to walk, and that she would have limited intelligence. Gertrude has survived cardiac arrests, lengthy surgical procedures, and complicated convalescences. Here she shares her memories of those years and the ways in which she has triumphed despite a medical history "as big as a football field."

CHAPTER 4

Struggling

by Gertrude Simpson

*T*his is the story of Gertrude Simpson, age 11, with a medical history as big as a football field. The stuff that I can remember begins when I was about 2 1/2 years old. I was in a room having some sort of a test. I was crying. The doctor tried to cheer me up. His name was Dr. Coldt. I thought of him as some kind of snowman because his name was Coldt. And there was Dr. Burger. I thought of him as Mr. Hamburger. There is one more—Dr. William. One day I needed x-rays and I was on the table. Dr. William and my mom were both wearing blue x-ray spacesuits. Suddenly out of the blue, I called him Dr. Dummy. He is one of the most important and strict doctors in the world, but surprisingly enough he liked it, and to this day he still does. I should also mention the nurses and doctors at home, like Lisa and Shirley and Dr. Johns and Linda Harrison. They are special.

Now back to the beginning. Dr. Coldt did a really good Donald Duck voice, or at least I thought so. He pulled out a Donald Duck puppet and made me laugh. The thing that made me remember this so well is that out of all the doctors in history, barely any of them can make a joke. I think that doctors should make jokes because it makes you feel a little more secure around your doctor.

The next thing that I remember was being in the hospital for 14 weeks. When I first came on the unit, we opened two blue swinging doors with chicken wire on the windows. We walked in the doors and there was an empty bed on the left side of the doors. I remember nurses named Fran and Patty who met us at the door. Patty was wearing blue surgery clothes and something to cover her hair. Patty has played a big role in my hospital life, but I'll write about her later. I have a perfect picture of the hospital room in my mind even though I was only 2 1/2 years old. I was in the last bed on the left. There were some kids across from me on beds. Next to them were two brown doors. If you entered those, you would go into the unit lobby. There were also doors across the room on the wide side of the room. One of the few things that I remember about Division 14 was the green, wet, buttery beans. We all had a window by our bed. I would always eat my green beans sitting cross-legged by my window. And another thing: I have always hated cold ice cream. The hospital always used to serve me ice cream. Since I hated it cold, Karen, my primary nurse, would take the ice cream and put it on the sunny window sill to turn it into "ice cream soup."

Since ice cream was a very important possession to me, I would have Karen put the ice cream in the freezer for my sister so that she could eat it when she came to visit. Sometimes the ice cream would sit in the freezer for 2 weeks at a time, because she didn't visit often. She lived too far away.

There is a jukebox in the hospital lobby. I would always play "Puff, the Magic Dragon." My first really clear memories of the hospital are from when I was 8 years old. I was in my sister's room at home and we were making bracelets. My mom and dad asked me to come downstairs. I sat on the couch, and my mom told me that I was going to have more surgery. They thought I was going to be depressed about going back to North East Children's Hospital, so they held back from telling me at first. But I was fine with it because I honestly didn't care. What I *really* wanted was to get my ears pierced, but I didn't want to go through the pain. So I wrote Dr. William and asked if he would pierce my ears while I was in surgery. He called me back and said yes.

The next part that I can remember is when I was going in for anesthesia. I was wheeled on the bed to the operating room. I looked around, asking what everything was. I wasn't scared because Patty, the nurse that I mentioned earlier, was in there with me. I had made special arrangements for her to be in the surgery room with me while they put me to sleep. They put the mask on and I didn't feel anything except the disgusting smell of the watermelon medicine. As I slowly drifted off I started to get pins and needles all over my body. This is really annoying because you have to lie perfectly still. Then I couldn't feel the lower half of my body. My sight slowly began to get less clear. My eyes weren't closed, so Patty told me I could close my eyes, which I did. I wanted to see what was happening, so I opened them again. When I did, I didn't see a normal thing. I saw the nurses in a black background with circles around their faces. Then I drifted off.

The next thing that I remember is when I was waking up. I tried to talk but I couldn't. I think that this is because you have a tube shoved down your throat and it is very sore. It's a little freaky because after being asleep for around 11 hours you want to talk to people. When I started to talk, the first thing I asked for was Patty, my special nurse. The nurses always shove air in your throat while you are waking up, which is really painful and annoying. They don't stop. After that, I asked for a mirror to look at my ears. They were pierced and I liked that.

Next, I wanted a barf basin. They brought me up to the room and I felt better. As we were waiting for the elevator, my mom gave me an envelope of cards from my classmates. Some of them were pretty stupid, but most of them were cool. It kind of cheered me up, although I didn't need much cheering up because I was happy about my ears and being with my friends at the hospital.

As we took the elevator up to the room, I lay there and waited. Then we got into the room and I turned on the television. After about 15 minutes Karen from Division 14, who was my favorite and primary nurse, came to see me. Then a very nice person, Lynn, the play lady, visited me and introduced me to the unit. I guess I had known her before, but I didn't remember.

They wheeled my bed and me into the playroom to check it out. The playroom was pretty cool. And then back to my room, and that's all I remember of that first day.

I also remember the next surgery when I turned 9 years old. I wrote Dr. William and asked if he would give me a bellybutton for my birthday, because all I had on my stomach was a lot of scars. He said yes, and we scheduled the next surgery for the fall. My mom had heard about the Hospitality House Program so we tried out a guest house. The people's names were Angie and Tom. They are really, really, really nice people and made us feel at home while we waited to go to the hospital.

The day we arrived in town, we went to the pre-op clinic. That night when we did a medical procedure, I noticed this huge lump on my stomach. I asked my mom to come look at it. Since it was really sore, I took a bath. Afterward, it still hurt, so my mom and dad called Dr. William, and he said that he would check it out the next day. He said it was a cyst that was probably infected and he canceled the planned bellybutton surgery. He planned to take me into the operating room the next day to drain it and told my parents that I would be discharged within 24 hours. My dad decided to go home to take care of my sister, and we sent him home with most of our clothes and my toys so that our suitcases would be light and easy to manage on the flight back to Florida.

Before I left home, I had been working on a play, and I was not going to be able to get to the performances because of this surgery. So when the operation plans changed, I was happy because I would get home in time for the opening. But when I woke up from the cyst surgery, my surgeon said it had been a lot more difficult than anticipated and I would have to stay in the hospital for about 9 days. I remember going into the playroom and playing on Super Nintendo. The playroom made me forget how much #6 pain I was in because it was really fun. When it was time to go home, the nurse taught me how to pack the wound because it was deep in my body. Once I learned, I pretty much got the hang of it and we took the airplane home.

I waited 5 months for my next and last surgery. I can't remember much about it except that my friend, whose mom is a flight attendant, came and visited us in the hospital. He lives in Florida too. I was on a liquid diet in case they needed to operate on my stomach. He and I went to eat out together the day before surgery, but I couldn't eat. I felt like I was going to die of hunger! After he left, it was time for my surgery. I don't remember the beginning, but I do remember what happened after. My aunt sent me a Play-Doh set from Las Vegas. My roommate and I played with it and had a good time. (My mom says this happened 2 years earlier. Since I have had so many surgeries, I mix up what happened in my memory.)

A couple of times a year I get together with other kids who have had the same kinds #6 of surgery. It's fun because Erin, one of my best friends, is there. Erin has played an important role in my healing. We talk about stuff a lot and she has also visited me in the hospital. She's a very good friend because she has the same medical history as me and we understand each other.

I go to a camp with kids who have medical stuff. It wasn't that much fun this year, but one of my best friends was there. Kate has the exact same medical problems as me and is really my best friend. Whenever I go to Las Vegas to see my aunt, I also visit Kate. We do a lot of stuff together, like going to movies and the mall.

When something is painful or boring you never forget it. I think I remember all this stuff because they were both. I also mention friends a lot because friends play a huge role in my recovery. For instance, one of my other best friends, Leah, would visit me frequently when I was in the hospital. I think she helped me recover mentally by cheering me up.

I think that my play lady Lynn helped me by keeping me occupied and keeping my mind off the hospital. She let me play Super Nintendo for hours. I know this is normally a bad thing for kids, but it is good for me in the hospital.

Probably the worst time I had at the hospital was in February 1995. They wanted to test my nerves in a certain spot where they had done a lot of surgery to see if I had feeling and muscle control. My mom asked if they were going to use any needles. They said no—just electrodes. First, they took my temperature and did stuff, and then when I was ready for the test, they told me that there was going to be a shot. I started to refuse the test, but my mom made me do it, which I think was very evil of her, and stupid. I went on to have the test, and they showed me the needle. My mom got mad at them because they had said that they weren't going to use needles and hadn't explained that these electrodes were needles. As they put the needle in, I made a scream of pain because it was the most painful thing I ever felt. They kept doing it until the test was over, and I think that that was a very evil, pathetic, useless, and dumb test because the test that I had next proved the exact same thing without the pain.

I think parents should always listen to their kids, and if they refuse the test parents should not agree to do the test. They should start letting children be part of making the decisions at age 9 because they are able by that age to make good decisions. There was a doctor who would wake me up at five o'clock in the morning just to ask how I was doing. I said, "I was doing just fine until you came in here and woke me." I thought the guy looked like a chipmunk, so I put a sign on my door that said, "No chipmunks allowed until 8 A.M." He never came back early in the morning again.

Another time that I will never forget is when I was really hungry after a surgery and my mother said that I should not eat yet. The resident disagreed with her in front of me and told me that it would be okay. Five minutes later I threw up like crazy on that doctor! I think that doctors should listen to the parents in cases like this, because they know their kids better than anyone.

I think that the nurses should treat kids really nicely because then the kids will cooperate. They should respect what the patient says even if the patient is young. I also think that it's good that North East Children's Hospital will not do procedures unless the parents are there, if possible. It is really good to have parents sleep in the hospital room with children because it helps us feel more secure. It is important to let family and friends visit.

In conclusion, this story is my medical life. Some of it won't be super clear because I wasn't old enough to remember all the details. I am who I am today because my mom helped me through all these struggles.

CRITICAL-THINKING ACTIVITIES

1. Gertrude begins her account by saying that as an 11-year-old she has a medical history "as big as a football field." What is your sense of the ways in which her knowledge of this has affected her day-to-day life?

2. How has Gertrude's experience allowed her to feel that her health-care providers are her advocates?

Doc - pierce ears / (joke)   Jukebox in the hospital lobby
Primary Nurse - Karen saved ice-cream for sister
Play lady Lyn

3. Explain in detail and give examples of the importance that primary nursing and Gertrude's primary nurses in particular have had.

4. Taking Gertrude's instruction on the importance of humor for children, write a paper in which you explore laughter and humor as a legitimate therapeutic art in the care and healing of children.

5. In this account the importance of friendship and the understanding of friends are stressed. How do you understand the importance of this child's friends for her? Can you expand this knowledge to children in your care?

6. Gertrude talks about her experience of pain after surgery and ways that she is able to transcend that pain. What are these ways, and what do you deduce from your findings?

7. Gertrude mentions the importance of certain foods and their effect upon her. How would you take this knowledge into account for all your patients? What might the implications be?

8. Gertrude's parents, sister, and grandparents have been crucial in her life. Explore the many ways that she has called that to our attention.

9. Gertrude provides several examples of ways in which she has been able to become a part of her treatment and recovery. What are those examples, and how could you translate this knowledge to your care of children? Why is the empowerment of the child crucial?

10. Not all of Gertrude's memories are pleasant. She also recalls the worst time she had at the hospital, when she was given a test to discover if nerves had regenerated at the surgical site. This test was excruciatingly painful, and she actively protested the proceedings. Later she notes that this test was unnecessary and makes a strong plea for being part of the decision making even though she is a minor. Create a model for decision making for doctors, nurses, parents, and child in which all concerned have equal and appropriate participation.

Ellen Simpson

Ellen Simpson is a therapist with a background in social work. She works
with children and adolescents in hospitals, mental health clinics, and
neonatal intensive care units. She has been married to Gertrude's father,
Michael, for 20 years. They have two daughters, Gabrielle and Gertrude.

 Here she reveals the psychological effects of parenting a challenged
child and the maxims she has developed in order to give Gertrude a
healthy and normal young life.

CHAPTER 5

The Challenge

by Ellen Simpson

*T*he challenges began even before Gertrude was born, 11 years ago. The medical system was set up to make it difficult for us to understand the situation and learn the possibilities. When we heard that there was the likelihood of a birth defect, we had to search for information, arrange meetings, and plan appropriate care for our soon-to-be-born child. Luckily, we had a superb supportive network and the courage to ask questions and choose doctors with whom we felt comfortable—even when that meant disengaging chiefs of services and alienating those on whom we had been dependent.

What we discovered along our journey is that there are some exceptionally rational, creative, brave, and sincere medical professionals, and that competence is multifaceted and inclusive of a variety of different skills. We chose those whom we thought we could work with and who had been recognized as the most successful in their field. I have thought many times about the mothers who do not have the education, knowhow, or financial resources to travel to a major medical center.

After Gertrude's birth, the first challenge was to be allowed to hold her. We all know that babies need warm, motherly contact when they leave the womb. I was told that no one was allowed to hold her. I asked how the staff had managed to change her isolette sheets. When I was told that they had gently lifted her fragile body up high enough so that another nurse could yank out the dirty sheet and replace it with a clean sheet, I arranged that no one other than her father or I be there when her sheets were changed, even if that meant waking me up in the middle of the night. (The nurses got a bit angry at me one time when I refused to give her back to them immediately. Her monitor was not buzzing and she clearly looked calm and comforted by my maternal touch.)

The next challenge was to move her to a hospital that would be willing to work with us to give her comfort and dignity. Several days after her traumatic birth, and our traumatic interactions with the medical community, we had her flown to a doctor and a hospital that encouraged family input and involvement. The chief of surgery there went so far as to ask us all, including her grandparents, to be in agreement with the treatment plan. He also encouraged me to breast-feed her, which I did gladly for many years and through many hospital visits. (This included the time that she went into full arrest at home and my milk dried up for 7 weeks. I pumped on the unit's breast pump every 3 hours around the clock. I needed to feed her with donor breast milk to supplement my supply until my milk returned.) At this hospital our involvement was welcomed. Even our 2 1/2-year-old daughter, Gabrielle, was encouraged to participate in her newborn sister's treatment. As traumatic as the birth was for us as parents, Gabrielle adjusted as only a little child could and touched and poked at our new baby with abandon.

As Gabrielle understood it, she had a sister who was not strong yet and needed to grow in the hospital before coming home. I am sure she sensed our stress, but she also sensed that the medical system was inclusive of her and that we were all trying to preserve a normal life for her. Her grandparents often cared for her during this period, and she has treasured memories of her time with them.

When Gertrude was almost 1 1/2 years old, we transferred her with her surgeon's consent to another facility for the next stage in her treatment. Gabrielle was 4 years old and had maintained a healthy approach to her sister's medical condition. She had been allowed to participate in much of the care, and as a result, neither girl felt isolated or alone. To this day they have the same connectedness as other siblings have. Gabrielle viewed her sister as less fragile than we did, and we allowed the girls freedom in their play together. Gabrielle used the bars on her sister's hospital bed as a jungle gym and encouraged her sister to stand on her head for exercise. They managed this without tangling the medical tubes.

There have been times when the nurses discouraged such abandon—for example, when Gertrude positioned her bed as high as it could go and observed the unit from a great height, with legs hanging over the side and tubing stretched to the maximum. During that hospital visit, she seemed to like playing with the outer limits of this bed. One nurse allowed her to go to sleep with the bed folded up like a V, with her huddled in the middle.

When Gertrude was 2 1/2 years old she had major surgical reconstruction at North East Children's Hospital. At times the nurses created experiences of unique play for her. When she experienced postsurgical complications that turned an expected 2-week recovery into a 14-week stay on Division 14 (the parent participation unit), her very special and loving primary nurse, Karen, acknowledged our daughter's complaints that she would not be able to go to the beach. One day Karen and several of the other creative nurses appeared with a huge tub of water, put Gertrude in a swimsuit, and gave her an afternoon to remember. They also let me take her into the hospital garden where, when no hospital personnel were looking, Gertrude found her way into the fountain. When she was well enough, they encouraged us to take her on a pass to a nearby park with wading pool.

This was the same staff and hospital unit that set up a cot by Gertrude's bed for her sister. She flew in from Florida every other week to see Gertrude and me. The cot facilitated comfort and nap time. The unit staff assisted my husband and me to parent both kids in as normal a way as possible. Living in a hospital with your child for months, as we have, is an awful task, but it can be made much easier by medical professionals and staff who care not only about the child but also about the family—parents, siblings, and grandparents. Those units that respect and use the parent's expertise find that, in the end, the child flourishes and develops with fewer traumatic memories.

Our daughter is a great example of this. When it is time for the next hospital trip, I greet the preparations with anxiety and worry, but she looks forward to the trip with excitement about seeing old friends (medical personnel) and being in an atmosphere where she can be herself and not "the only one."

We are now working exclusively with the Children's Hospital medical team. We will remain there for the completion of treatment. When I am with the surgeon, Dr. Harry William, I feel as if I am experiencing an important moment in medical history.

He is recognized as one of the most successful in the world, having invented and perfected many of the operative procedures used in surgery today. Our daughter owes much of who she is to his competence. He has great compassion for the children he touches. He may be very busy in the operating room for up to 20 hours at a time, and he rarely sees a child post-op, but when Gertrude is with him, he is totally present for her. When she was 2 1/2, he never left her side during her 17-hour reconstructive surgery. I was embarrassed to admit that I fell asleep while he worked gently on my baby. He always has time to respect his patients. I have seen him get angry at residents and interns who did not treat families with the professionalism that he demands. I recognize that he intimidates some families and staff who work with him, but he demands excellence, and if he feels that you are not meeting that goal, he challenges you to do so.

Not only do I appreciate his precise surgical technique. I appreciate his sensitivity—in responding to the valentine our daughter sent him, in agreeing to pierce her ears, and in responding to her request for a bellybutton on her ninth birthday.

Many parents are fearful about asking questions. The doctors are frequently rushed or may not know the answer. It is important to compose a list before meeting with them and to ask until you have answers. We as consumer parents have a right not only to receive answers but to *understand*. So do our children. At what age do the kids need to be told what is happening? At Children's Hospital they encourage as much preparation as possible. At certain developmental stages, short notification was more appropriate for Gertrude; at other stages, she benefited from knowing the plan far in advance. Parents can best assess this for their own children with the help of people knowledgeable in child development and psychology. Our daughter thinks that by age 9 she was ready to make decisions about her medical care. I do not disagree. I think that it is important to involve children in appropriate decisions as early as possible. Encourage them to make choices when they can. For instance, if there is an option about which day they will undergo a painful procedure, let them choose. At this time in her life, Gertrude does not fear the hospital, except for the needles. She trusts that either her father or I will be with her at all times, that one of her favorite nurses will be with her during anesthesia induction, that we will be there when she wakes up, and that Dr. William will be with her the whole time she is in surgery and until it is safe for him to leave.

How do children maintain their dignity in the hospital? As I said, they should be given choices whenever possible. Their bodies should not be exposed unnecessarily. Cover them up with double robes and extra sheets, and pull the curtains for procedures. If strange nurses or doctors do not need to be in the room, ask them to leave until the procedure is completed. So what if they are studying—there are plenty of other opportunities for them to learn. If not, and they must be there, insist that they first establish a relationship with your child. There are very few crises in the recovery process that require the team to run in, pull back the sheets, and get to work without first introducing themselves. It can be quite simple: "Hi, I'm Dr. So-and-so. You must be Jimmy. Do you know why I am here? Today I am going to do this. Before we begin, what are your questions and concerns?" Both children and family members feel out of control so often in the hospital. But I have learned to maximize my coping skills and to adapt them to the hospital culture.

There are many ways for parents to protect their children in the hospital. It is equally important, when the time is right, to maintain healthy discipline for hospitalized children. My daughter disagrees and thinks that hospitalization is not the time for the unenjoyable routines of life. She thinks that recovery is dependent on the amount of pleasurable activities allowed per day (television, Super Nintendo, arts and crafts). I actually agree with her that she recovers more rapidly when afforded the opportunity to enjoy herself and to be distracted from pain and immobility. I wish that she agreed with me that healing is also dependent on the reestablishment of her normal daily lifestyle. I want her to recognize that she is not so debilitated that we are going to allow her to regress: Life continues even under the difficult circumstances of prolonged hospital stays. My goal has always been to create as regular an atmosphere as possible, within the context of a lot of nonhealth.

I have often wondered if the staff on the unit has any idea how important information becomes to parents. When you see the doctors only once a day (if you are lucky and happen to catch them on rounds), every word they say about recovery and discharge becomes significantly magnified. When the resident states that "we are *hoping* to stop the IV this morning," I wonder why it's still in at 10. A.M. No matter how often I have been with her in the hospital, I still get foolishly invested in the daily pronouncements of progress. I should have learned by now that nothing is final until the surgeon has said it directly to me, but I remain so anxious for information that I believe what others say. I also try to figure out information from what they are not saying—tests results that are not given to us, body language, and moods.

Did the residents who had never treated my daughter before have any comprehension of the situation they created by telling me that she would be discharged in 2 days? Knowing that she has usually developed some difficulties on day 3 or 4, but valuing all possibilities of rapid discharge, I foolishly believed what they said. And then I panicked. I feared flying home with her so soon—far away from Children's Hospital. I arranged to stay in town for a week, and my husband and I discussed the possibilities of rehospitalization, insurance coverage, etc. Later that evening, the surgeon visited and was as shocked as I was at this plan. The next night she started bleeding and by the next morning, they were discussing bringing her back into the operating room. It is good that I was still in town, and better yet that she was still in the hospital.

When children live in hospitals as much as Gertrude has, the transition to home life can be difficult. After weeks of continual invasion by nurses and doctors, and the noise of monitors, you have the much-needed quiet and privacy of home. This is usually mixed with feelings of elation and depression. Separation from the hospital can be quite scary at first. The need for continued medical procedures and dressing changes and exercises and strong medications with numerous side effects—suddenly you have no one to whom you can go with questions. We are so far away from the hospital that once we have left, we do not return for months. The medical isolation at home can overwhelm both Gertrude and me, and we have to structure things so that we feel comfortable with the medical tasks.

Returning to school is frequently even more traumatic than returning to the hospital. Suddenly the child is thrust back into a normal world yet is still required to undergo unusual medical procedures. People act as if things were regular for her, as if the worst were over, when in fact it has taken as much as 6 post-operative weeks for Gertrude to get back into her normal routine. With each discharge I become better at helping her make the transition. I have never been offered help by the medical community in this very sensitive area of her healing and recovery. Sometimes there are disadvantages to appearing competent. Since we have been so successful at helping our daughter thrive against great odds, medical professionals think that we are extremely capable and do not offer assistance, like visiting nurses. Sure, we can hire a nurse privately, but that becomes exceedingly expensive.

It's odd that health insurance readily pays for inpatient but not for outpatient treatment. There was a situation several years ago when she needed IV medication. If administered in the hospital, the cost would be nothing to us but $10,000 to the insurance company. If it was administered at home, the cost would have been family stability and $3,000 to us, and nothing to the insurance company. We felt it was important to keep her out of the hospital for emotional reasons, but we knew that the cost would put a significant strain on our resources. The doctor was willing to do whatever we chose. Through a lot of creativity and flexibility on the part of our pediatrician, my husband negotiated with the insurance company to make special arrangements to fund the IV at home. They saved themselves $7,000, we did not have to put her in the hospital, and everyone was happier.

I think the constant noises and smells of the hospital affect parents and their ability to think clearly. People tell you to go out for a break, but, so frequently, you return to some minor crisis and feel guilty for having left your child unsupervised. If possible, I leave only when assured that a friend or relative will stay with my child and protect her from unnecessary pain or stress.

Several years ago, I left to go to the bank and when I returned I discovered that a volunteer had brought some lovely Mylar balloons to my daughter. Then why was she in tears? The balloons were tied to a latex balloon that was filled with pebbles and used as a colorful weight. Gertrude is severely allergic to latex, there are precautions written all around her room, and this innocent mistake caused her panic. Things like this happen. They do not seem so great to the casual observer. However, mistakes take on a bigger significance when she is feeling vulnerable. When hooked up to IVs and not allowed to get out of bed, a child's power and sense of competence diminishes. To her, that small latex balloon was massive. She still speaks with fear and a feeling of abandonment when remembering the time that she was brought chicken broth while I was in the shower. It was placed on her tray in front of her, and she was handed a spoon. She was lying prone and immobile, but she was hungry so she tried to manage and ended up spilling "burning" soup all over herself. How do children feed themselves when they do not have attentive parents?

Children on surgical units are not "appendectomies," "craniofacial repairs," or "spina bifidas." They are small people with medical needs. Their diagnoses do not define them, nor do their procedures explain them. They need to be honored for the individuals that they are and treated with respect. So do their parents. How difficult it is to sleep in a room with crying strangers night after night and be expected to wake up looking and acting like a competent consumer of medical services. Does it ever occur to the resident that he or she was not the only one up all night worrying? I really don't want to be told their problems of exhaustation when I am feeling similarly, nor do I even care. I expect them to behave as if my child is the most important child in the hospital at that moment. I ask that they be honest about my daughter's condition and save the condescension for others. And if they do not know the answer to my question, find it out!

Over the past 11 years I have developed coping skills for the inpatient stays. It's unfortunate but true that if I present myself as a competent and attractive woman, they treat me better. My trick: Shower every morning and dress as if I am going to work. Be ready to greet the earliest of the shifts, and have questions prepared for rounds. Never let my frustration get out of control in front of the staff (save it for phone calls with my husband at night), and always defend Gertrude's rights and needs, even at the risk of alienating someone. Find out who on the unit is child-centered, and surround your child with those staff. When things get really tense, leave—but always take your child if you can. I try to develop relationships with other parents that are mutually rewarding and reciprocal. We have learned to seek out only those parents who energize and strengthen us—and we try to reciprocate.

What is it like to live for years with the fear of sudden death or illness? I know that this has had a profound impact on me. We can rarely predict when a crisis is coming, but we always have to be prepared. I kept a suitcase packed for years, just in case I had to fly off suddenly to the hospital with her. I never felt that I could plan for an activity without a backup plan for sickness. We appreciate the healthy, pain-free days in a way that no one can comprehend without witnessing the nights of agony and distress. Only recently was I brave enough to ask the doctor if she would have a normal life expectancy. The answer is yes.

Gertrude is just coming into the belief that she is now strong—in some ways bionic. When her grandfather suddenly died last year, she stated that she had always thought that she would be the first one to die in the family. So now we have a new task. Helping her to believe that she is going to be here for many years to come, and helping her through the normal challenges of adolescence. Perhaps that will be more difficult than any of those nights in the hospital.

CRITICAL-THINKING ACTIVITIES

1. The author has described several ways in which she and her husband "mobilized resources" when they learned that their second child would be born prematurely. Explain exactly what these parents did and how their actions have affected their lives and the lives of their children.

2. Ellen Simpson believed it was very important to hold her frail, premature infant in the NICU. Do you agree? How would you support this parental involvement in your future practice? Discuss in detail.

3. Using examples from this narrative, explain the central role of the relationship between Gertrude and her sister, Gabrielle. How might you, as a health-care professional, support and encourage sibling relationships?

4. Discuss the ways in which the accessibility of this family has influenced Gertrude's welfare and recovery.

5. Karen and other nurses provided Gertrude with a "day at the beach" in her hospital room. This creative act of play and laughter enjoyed by the child and others around her most certainly had an effect on her recovery by counteracting disappointment and discouragement. How, exactly, do such powerful emotions affect somatic responses?

6. Ellen Simpson has learned that normal, healthy discipline is crucial, even though her child is ill and in pain. Discuss what this reestablishment of daily routine and school work might accomplish. Include ways in which you could support parents in this endeavor.

7. What are your ethical guidelines for sharing information with parents and children? What is the basis for them?

8. Develop a model of care for the guidance of children reentering home life and school after long hospitalizations. Take into consideration the continued need for medical and nursing involvement owing to healing wounds and so forth.

9. What exactly does the author wish to have residents, interns, and nurses know about their professional discipline when they are involved with parents and children? Why is this so crucial to our understanding?

10. What does the author suggest that parents do to advocate for themselves and for their children? Concentrate especially on her advice for managing controversy and tension. Why are her points important to note?

Christopher Edwards

Christopher Edwards is a writer, editor, and publishing consultant. His published works include *Crazy for God* (Prentice-Hall, 1979) and *Entrepreneurial Science* (Quorum, 1987). He is the founding editor-in-chief of *Bio Technology* magazine and has been a consulting editor for Random House, Macmillan, McGraw-Hill, and other publishers. Edwards completed a BA in psychology and philosophy at Yale University, pursued graduate work in theology at Princeton Seminary, and is working on a PhD in philosophy and literature at Boston University.

In his account of his childhood, Edward reveals "terror that has spilled over into three major hospitalizations and three marriages." He vividly describes what fostered his recovery and what actually hurt him. His experience is distilled in a poignant poem, "The Wounding."

CHAPTER 6

Understand

by Christopher Edwards

I grew up in a vicious greenhouse, the kind of place that was sufficiently remote from outside predators, famine, and disease to win the envy of the workmen who came to fix the plumbing and rake the leaves. The words "privileged" and "molded" come to mind, as well as the word "formulaic," descriptors for a life intended to make me the object of family pride. In fact, this greenhouse was a glass prison. I was unprotected and invisible, except when needed. Subjected to attacks from an older brother who tried to kill me because I had two legs and he had one. Overseen by an elderly fundamentalist grandmother who screamed of the doom of Cain and Abel when my brother and I battled. Ignored by a mother who survived breast cancer shortly after my birth but predicted her death daily between doses of phenobarbital. And shaped by a father who asserted himself by saying things like, "Just remember, I could destroy you," to his little boys. So I was a good boy—as good as I could be—but rarely me.

As I approach my 42nd year, I feel gratitude for the women and men who have helped me through my recovery from the terror of my childhood, terror that has spilled over into three major hospitalizations and three marriages. I also remain bitter about the therapists who took my money without helping me or, in several instances (always with psychiatrists), actually abused me. I want to tell you about what actually worked and what really hurt me.

What worked is ridiculously simple, so simple that it's a shame to have to state it. The turning points during all of my psychoses have occurred when people dared to enter my world, reflected my experience back to me with empathy (but not necessarily agreement), and offered me choices. In one case, I moved toward sanity and out of the hospital after conversations with a chaplain and a volunteer. Both in their own ways took my dilemmas and my story—as I saw them and described them—very seriously. In understanding me without humoring me, they somehow helped me to believe in myself and to believe that I could stitch myself back together again. They listened as if my stories were true, if only just for me. And so I had permission to be sane again, to return to that common set of beliefs about the world that we all share in the daily rubbings and drubbings of our lives.

In another instance, I started my turn toward sanity after convincing my wife to become my court-appointed trustee and then to overrule the hospital's decisions. The administration had wanted to send me to a state institution for a minimum of 3 months,

49

since I wasn't responding to the doctors' cocktails. My dishonorable discharge, complete with signed papers and disclaimers on the hospital's part, was made possible because my wife believed me and involved me in my own fate once again. I felt safe to take control over my life and eventually returned home with some degree of stability.

Another of my hospitalizations ended when my father simply came up to me and said, "Your Blue Cross coverage here is over. You can stay on, but it will be very expensive. Or you can come home with me and stay with us for a while." It was the first time during a 5-week hospitalization when I was offered a choice about something.

What hasn't worked? When therapists and institutions relied too heavily on medications, assuming that basic maintenance and waiting for the biochemical magic to take effect were enough. When nobody took the time to share my world with me and bring me into theirs. When the closest thing to human interaction was the drone of a television set, constantly tuned to one station while the staff invisibly performed their institutional duties. When hospitals, modeled after prisons in so many respects, focused more on their own efficiency than on their healing missions.

How can a person heal in a place where strangers are constantly screaming and floating down the halls in medicated states, where basics like access to sunlight and soothing sounds are nonexistent, where nurses have time only to push carts down the hall, dispensing "meds" like stewardesses passing out whiskey and peanuts to passengers during a crowded airline flight? How many times have I seen attendants spend more time with their newspapers and bestsellers than with the patients themselves? I strongly believe that the minimization of real human contact negated the positive effects of medications during my hospitalizations. One reason for this lack of contact is clear. Too often I have encountered mental health workers in institutions who seem to be afraid of "the crazy people," turning them into objects by ignoring them, laughing at them, or talking about them to other workers. Patients hear and often understand, and they hurt too much and too easily.

The issue of listening to patients brings to mind another point. The stories of "crazy people" need to be taken as expressions of the creative self in the making. In my case, my moments of psychotic madness were attempts to create a self that was both deeply personal and fully connected to other people. Paradoxically, I did this by creating, entering into, and believing a fictional world that became a psychological refuge. My delusions were not symptomatic of a loss of self but were signs of the struggle to recreate a self in a livable way. Much as a fiction writer superimposes his own life experiences upon fictional characters to give his struggles shape and meaning from a distance, the delusions I have expressed and heard from many others took on this distant, secondary, but crucial life for the patient. If you take the time to seriously listen to delusions instead of treating them simply as artifacts of a miswired brain, you can decipher and help to treat a struggling patient. Although the stories aren't real, the feelings behind the stories *are*. And sometimes it is possible to connect to the feeling self only through the avenues of the delusions, the departures from the seen. This route has worked well for me in my maddest moments as well as during the more stable times of my treatment.

I have observed the importance of such fictional engagements when trying to help someone who is very dear to me, my wife. I stayed with her over several days during two manic episodes within a 2-month interval. She seemed to be evolving a language to speak about aspirations and dreams that she was never allowed to have. I grew to see her manic episodes as creative events, the first as a birth event, the second as that of a child learning how to use art and the tools of language in deciding to assert herself as an individual, expressive being. In seeing such episodes as evidence of uneven growth in a person instead of pathology, I could understand her better and support her as she strove to actualize those psychotically experienced ambitions within the constraints and possibilities of the real world. Because of her courageous efforts, she has emerged as a happier and more stable person.

I want to finish by underscoring my claim that the stories of the mentally ill are worth exploring. The following poem was written a few weeks after my last hospitalization. Looking at it 5 years later, I remember that I wrote it while in the early stages of recovery, when I was unable to function in everyday life. I include it here to illustrate the continuity between the fictions of the delusional self and the road it maps out for recovery into a saner and more reflective version of the emerging person.

While experiencing my psychoses in the hospital, I tried to wound myself in what I considered to be an imitation of and obedience to Christ. I literally believed and replayed the roles and events I later symbolized in this poem. Returning from the hospital, I interpreted my psychotic experiences and the hospitalization as a painful but necessary type of spiritual awakening, hence a wounding of a different order. The allusion in the poem to a prisoner on death row awaiting electrocution reminded me of my experience of life on earth as a sentence that would be commuted only by death. The extended arms of the Christ-friend inviting me to a sweet afterlife symbolized the resurgence of my Christian faith through the pain of psychoses and hospitalization.

I now connect both the original delusion and the subsequent interpretations to my imprisonment in a "vicious greenhouse" as a child, my abandonment by my mother, and my willingness to hurt myself and anticipate being hurt by my father and brother in order to earn love. And I also hear the echoes of my fundamentalist grandmother urging me to be good or to suffer the fate of Cain and Abel.

THE WOUNDING

Come cry for us all
The lonely in prison
Who rattle our feeble cups and our trays
Against the arms of those awful gates
Hoping for kindness in eyes upon us
That watch the drool on our pillows collect
And count the cracks in our sorry feet

Hold me in this womb of iron
And keep my toes on the soft slab floor
While the well-to-do sip espresso
And boast of their children's new homes

My child is dreaming for me
When I look in the mirror
He turns in shame
My wife is so tired of lawyers
She fans her sweat with the warden's reports

I hear the sting of the chair next door
And the pacing of friends
Who wait their turn
This wood I claim
Will singe my wrists
As the arms of my best friend extend
He shouts
My palace of sorrows is waiting for you

So cry for us all
Love moistens my cheek
A hymn rides my breath when I sigh
Be sure when you cry in joy to pray
That you may be wounded like this one day.

—Chris Edwards

CRITICAL-THINKING ACTIVITIES

1. Chris Edwards believes that certain actions that fall under the rubric of mental health care actually hurt patients. What examples does he give? Why are these actions harmful?

2. Why does the author insist that those suffering from mental illness should have the experience of sunlight and soothing sounds? How could you implement these experiences in your setting?

3. Why is it important to realize that psychotropic medications are not a cure-all? How does Edwards view these drugs? What is their appropriate place in the treatment of mental illness?

4. What are psychotic delusions? How would you approach someone who is experiencing delusions? Are the author's suggestions for a creative approach viable? Discuss in full.

5. The behavior of the psychiatrists, nurses, mental health workers, and other patients in this narrative seem quite similar to key figures in the author's life. Explore the implications of these similarities.

6. How would you suggest reorganizing inpatient psychiatric care to avoid the hurtful actions noted in this account?

7. Discuss the ways in which mental health professionals suffer from habits of mind and systems of beliefs similar to those described by Allan H. Macurdy in Chapter 2?

8. How is the author's experience distilled in "The Wounding"?

Donna Griesenbeck

Donna Griesenbeck earned a BA in German and an MA in Russian and has lived and studied extensively in Europe and Russia. She is an interpreter and translator and now works in the Slavic language program at Harvard University.

She enjoys choral singing, cooking, walking, bicycling, and volunteering for an organization that teaches self-defense.

Here she chronicles her 6-year struggle with bipolar disorder and shares her discovery: Examining links and parallels between her psychosis and everyday struggles as one might examine a work of art has helped her to heal and to explore new avenues for subsequent development.

CHAPTER 7

Psychosis: Art, Life, or Illness?

by Donna Griesenbeck

Six years ago I was diagnosed with bipolar disorder (manic-depressive illness). I see two major phases of my struggle with bipolar disorder: the first involved grappling with the initial psychotic experiences and resulting diagnosis; and once the disorder had been brought more or less under control, the next phase was dealing with nagging issues like drug side effects, stigmatization, and doubts about the diagnosis. Compared with others who have this disorder, I have confronted relatively few hurdles as I come to terms with the disease. My family and friends have been understanding and supportive. My three hospitalizations have been relatively brief (under 2 weeks each) and have not caused repercussions in the workplace. My health insurance has covered all my hospitalization costs and paid for significant work in therapy. And fortunately, during my manic episodes I never did anything that caused either physical or financial damage.

Despite all these advantages, adapting to and learning to live with bipolar disorder has been a difficult and often painful experience. But my struggle with the disorder, particularly during the first phase, has resulted in personal growth on a more dramatic level than I might otherwise have achieved in these past 6 years. I would like to offer a vignette of this struggle and how it has helped me to mature, followed by a brief discussion of some of the more mundane issues that appear to be a permanent part of life with this illness.

My first manic episode took place when I was in my late twenties. The small academic institute where I worked was in its final days, but we were still fighting and hoping for a reprieve. Late at night on the day the definitive closing announcement was made, I awoke from a half-slumber with the sudden inspiration to write a book that would connect all the people I cared about in one beautiful, intricate web. I called my parents and excitedly shared this news. Soon after hanging up I had a strong premonition that I was about to die and that my mother would write the book instead. I wrote a will and called some people I loved to give them advance notice and ensure that they would not feel pangs of guilt over not having contacted me recently. Toward morning I had a strange experience in which I felt like I was being physically reborn; I actually felt the birth contractions massaging my body. I emerged with the conviction that I had just been born as an artist.

That day I had lucid spells alternating with visions illustrating the interconnectedness of all beings and other, less easily articulated spiritual insights. I felt I possessed a unique spiritual understanding that I was to communicate to others. At last I had a calling in life, and it would be quite literally a "calling"—I believed I was destined to live out my days waiting for calls or letters inviting me to work, travel, or simply spend time with people. I would be free from the need to make any decisions at all; I was merely to respond to all invitations in the affirmative.

By late that night these visions had more or less ceased, and I found myself wandering through the kitchen, knowing I needed to eat but unable to choose anything. Being in this state of utter indecision about an elementary bodily function made me realize that I needed help. My roommates took me to the emergency room, where I spent the remainder of the night. When I arrived there, I was nearly catatonic and found myself unable to carry out the requests of the emergency room staff. I perceived great hostility on their part and recall being taunted and threatened with catheterization if I could not produce a urine sample. Whether their hostility was real or imaginary, it aroused in me the belief that these people were the spiritual dregs of the earth and that they were in the process of crucifying me. I was doomed to wait on the cross while history rewound itself like a film and then played itself out as it should have been the first time around: a sort of retroactive redemption. Only after the process was complete could I rejoin the rest of creation. Around the time I expected to be lifted from the cross, I was taken to a psychiatric hospital. At first, I believed the hospital to be paradise, a place where I had been reunited with everyone I loved and cared about. Later, when I was under the influence of Haldol and other drugs, the bleak reality made itself known to me. By the time I was discharged, I felt physically weak, shaky, lethargic, and deeply depressed.

The several months that followed were far more difficult than anything I have faced since. I was having severe side effects from the Haldol and did not respond well to the usual "sidecar" medications. My psychiatrist seemed to ignore my complaints and offered little hope that I would ever feel better. After a couple of months, he broke the news of my diagnosis to me by handing me a booklet about lithium therapy and saying, "Read this. You'd better get used to it." Previously, he had never even suggested to me that I had a mental illness. My assumption was that I had had a "nervous breakdown" or some other acute attack, but I believed that things would settle down and return to normal. When I read the booklet, I did not recognize myself in the profile of a bipolar-disorder patient. I resisted accepting the diagnosis and opposed any drug treatment, in part because my experience with Haldol had confirmed my prejudice against psychiatric drugs in general. When, in desperation, I took matters into my own hands and announced to my psychiatrist that I planned to stop taking Haldol, he told me cockily, "You'll be back." He was right: After a few days of a euphoric "like myself again" feeling, I began to have bouts of anxiety and insomnia.

Fearing another psychotic episode, I returned to my health maintenance organization but requested and met with another psychiatrist. The contrast in manner between the two psychiatrists was striking. This one sat me down, described the symptoms that had been observed in me, stated that they fit the diagnosis of bipolar disorder, and then presented me with several options, one of which was simply to monitor my progress without any drug treatment at all. As we discussed the options and their likely outcomes, I became more open to the idea of lithium therapy and made the conscious, informed decision to try it. This exchange marked the beginning of a supportive, empathetic patient-doctor relationship that saw me through a period of sustained good health.

In retrospect, I see that I could have used an advocate to tell me that I had the right to a doctor with whom I felt comfortable and who was responsive to my needs. It took me several months to muster the courage to assert this right on my own, and I would have benefited from proper care right from the start. But in a depressed state and with no prior experience with mental health care, I had no idea what my rights were.

At the same time that I began lithium therapy, I also started seeing a therapist who was extremely helpful in managing the emotional issues that accompanied my illness, diagnosis, and treatment. Denial was a major issue for me. In certain phases I would view my psychosis as a symptom or expression of emotional turmoil, instead of a sign of an underlying biochemical problem. My therapist would acknowledge the links and parallels between my psychosis and my everyday struggles, then gently voice her belief that biochemical or other physical factors also played a crucial role. Without ridiculing or devaluing my interpretations of my psychotic episodes, she motivated me to adhere to my lithium treatment plan. In this relationship, too, I felt I was being presented options and could choose among them for myself.

My therapist's affirmation of the personal meaning I could find in my psychotic episodes has encouraged me to explore my memories for clues to my underlying spiritual, psychological, and emotional issues. In my experience, psychosis has both reflected my current state and foreshadowed my future personal development and healing. By examining my memories of the psychosis as I would a work of art, I have been able to identify emotional issues that I still need to address.

For example, in the psychotic experience described above, some of the personal issues I see expressed are a too-strong "other" orientation, fear of decision making, repression of my creativity, and a tendency to withdraw into religiosity. I do not believe that the memories of psychosis alone brought these problems to my awareness; on the contrary, usually I would recognize a pertinent issue during a therapy session and later see how certain pieces of the psychosis expressed it in a powerful and highly individual way. When I am able to make sense of my bizarre memories, the achievement is reminiscent of the satisfaction I once felt in college upon identifying a meaningful pattern in a work of literature. In addition, each new meaning I am able to discern in my psychotic experience is an index of my increased self-awareness.

At the same time, certain images have challenged me to explore new avenues for subsequent development. The image of life as a work of art, and myself as an artist, was a major theme of my first psychotic episode. The midwife for my birth as an artist was someone I had phoned on the first night of my psychosis, the mother of the family I had lived with for a year as an exchange student. This is a family of extraordinarily creative art professionals, and my year with them had opened my eyes to a whole new way of living. The image of being born as an artist perfectly expresses the significance of this family, particularly the mother, for me. Since the psychotic episode I have become more and more mindful of my need to develop and express my creativity. I still would not use the word "artist" to describe myself, but I am learning to view myself as a creative person. During my psychosis I had a vivid experience of the joy of inspiration and creativity, and the memory of it has motivated me to allow my creativity to flow more freely in my everyday life.

It is vitally important to allow individuals to draw their own conclusions about their psychotic experiences. Stereotypes and generalizations ("delusions of grandeur," "flights of fancy") ignore the uniquely individual meaning that the psychotic experience expresses. To illustrate, when I requested and read a copy of my psychiatric record, I found a notation that I had believed myself to be Jesus Christ. This was an utter misunderstanding of my experience. I had described the sensation of undergoing a crucifixion at the hands of the emergency room staff, but at no time had I believed myself to be

Jesus. Looking back on the events surrounding that first episode, I realized that I had felt like a martyr in my job. What more powerful metaphor of martyrdom could a well-churched mind conjure up in a state of psychosis? Or in a lucid state, for that matter? It was a magnification, perhaps an exaggeration, of what I felt, but it expressed something that I was either unaware of or unable to express in other ways.

In spite of lithium therapy, I have had three manic episodes since the first one. The themes of spirituality, friends and family, and creativity have been central to all my psychotic experiences. I can, however, identify a progression from a strict church-bound religiosity toward a broader spirituality, a progression that parallels my personal development over the same period. My behavior in each subsequent episode has also become successively more active and autonomous, and my area of concerns more down-to-earth. Whether this "taming" of the psychotic experience has been due to continued lithium (now supplemented with Depakote) therapy, earlier intervention, my considerable personal development, or all three, I am not likely ever to find out. Whatever the underlying biophysical reality, I am convinced that the suppression of my creative and spiritual self also contributed to my experiences of psychosis. By integrating the interpretation of my psychotic experiences into my everyday life, I am able to reclaim neglected aspects of my authentic self. As I more consciously develop my creativity, I believe that I lessen the likelihood and the severity of another episode.

The experiences I have described illustrate how the challenge of altering my self-concept to integrate my experiences with mental illness led to significant personal growth. Now that I have settled into a treatment regime and attained a so-called normal routine, other, more mundane issues have come into play.

I still have side effects from the lithium, but I have found ways to manage. Hand tremors are the most annoying side effect, and they are usually a problem only when I am nervous. In social situations where a mishap would be especially embarrassing (for example, while eating soup or drinking from a full glass or cup) the tremors become severe, almost spasmodic. Now I take propranolol before anxiety-provoking events like lunch meetings and job interviews, and this helps enormously. I should mention that the first time I experienced severe tremors, I was leading a tour group in what was then the Soviet Union. I thought I was having lithium toxicity and lowered my dose. Two days later I was in the throes of a full-blown psychotic episode and wound up in a mental hospital. If I had known about propranolol before that trip, I might have been spared that hospitalization. Lately, I have begun to develop some control over the tremors by reminding myself that if I can lift a half-full cup of coffee to my lips without shaking, why not a full or even over-full cup?

Perhaps the most disturbing aspect of life with bipolar disorder is the feeling that it must be kept secret. I feel that I would be overstepping the bounds of normal social behavior if I were to reveal my condition to anyone but my closest friends. I confront this issue on a regular basis in my job, which does not use my best skills but is relatively pleasant and secure. I have predictable hours; good, cheap health insurance; and sympathetic coworkers and supervisors. I constantly vacillate between wanting to venture forth and seek more fulfilling work and wanting to play it safe and make do with what I have. Occasionally people ask me how long I plan to stay in my job, or what I want to do next (subtext: "You can't possibly be planning to work here indefinitely!"), and I feel I have to concoct believable excuses for staying put. Even if to some degree I am projecting my own judgments onto the people who ask, I know that the basic sentiment is there. If I had my way, I would tell anyone who inquired about my career ambitions that I remain in a less-than-satisfying job because of the security it offers, and that I need the security to manage my life with bipolar disorder. I want an airtight excuse for what I perceive as my failure to make better use of my talents and education.

I should point out that, as far as I understand, there is actually no physical reason relating to bipolar disorder that should prevent me from tackling more challenging work. And I am fully aware that many jobs offer benefits, some even better than what I have. Yet I cling to the security of the job I know because I fear destabilization. I feel safe in this job because I know I will not be fired or ostracized if, God forbid, I were to have another manic episode. I could never know for certain whether this would be true in another work situation.

An additional frustration of not being able to be open about my experiences with bipolar disorder comes from the knowledge that my silence perpetuates the stereotypes about mental illness—the very stereotypes I fear will be applied to me. The idea that you can "tell" if someone has a mental illness has come out again and again when I take the risk and reveal my experience to someone. Virtually without exception, the response is something like, "I never would have guessed," which leads me to wonder how many other people there must be who have a mental illness that you'd never suspect. This brings home to me how great the need is to educate people about mental illness.

I continue to have periodic doubts about the diagnosis and its basis in physiological reality. Because I am able to make sense of much of what I experienced during psychosis, it raises the question of whether I really have a biological disorder at all or if I have experienced what some psychologists have called "spiritual crises." My recent reading has included works that challenge the existing models of mental illness and psychotherapy, charging that they fail to take into account the vast range of experience that transcends the strictly personal. These works raise the question of where and how to draw the line between "normal" and "abnormal." Although I believe my work in therapy has, on the whole, encouraged my self-acceptance and expression, I still wonder at times if the focus on coping and leading a "normal" life may cause me to avoid the riskier path of greater individuality.

The prevailing notion that there is a high correlation between manic depression and creative genius occasionally causes me difficulty. I would like nothing better than to have the gift of powerful artistic expression. That would give me another justification for my low career achievement: I would then be working a "day job" to support my artistic mission. Unfortunately, I have no artistic mission. I work my day job and do a variety of activities that could be considered creative, but I have nothing resembling an artistic mission. Instead of expressing my individuality, I feel I must hide what has been the central fact of my existence over the past 6 years: my struggle to cope with bipolar disorder.

CRITICAL-THINKING ACTIVITIES

1. How did the emergency room staff's inability to understand the author's immobility heighten her fears and result in a worsening of her condition?

2. How did this episode manifest itself in the medical record? How could this lack of understanding and subsequent misinterpretation of a patient's statement influence diagnosis and treatment?

3. Discuss the ways in which the first psychiatrist's conduct negatively influenced the author.

4. Design a model for collaboratively conducting lithium therapy. Take into consideration the second psychiatrist's methods, the realistic experience of possible side effects, and the implications of long-term medication for a chronic illness.

5. What is your understanding of the way in which the author and her therapist approach the integration of her psychosis with everyday past and present struggles? Give examples from the narrative.

6. How has this author shown us that an individual's range of experiences transcends the personal?

7. Explore Ms. Griesenbeck's contribution to the dispelling of the stigma of mental illness.

Greg Lum

Greg Lum, a native of San Francisco, graduated from the University of California at Berkeley. He attained an MA at New York University and is presently at work on a doctoral dissertation at Boston University on the subject of dramatic adaptation of classical works of literature. Having returned to his home in San Francisco, he teaches English in the public school system.

Seven years ago while crossing a street he was hit by a car speeding in a school zone. This event began his experience with chronic pain, which is the subject of his account.

CHAPTER 8

Prisoner of Pain

by Greg Lum

I suppose I can consider what being in pain is like by looking at how the pain has affected the way I live my life. But first, I'd like to consider the problem of even describing pain—specifically, what pain is like for me, how chronic pain appears, how it feels, and how it affects me psychologically and emotionally. Especially important is the issue of being in control.

For some, chronic pain is merely a long-term sentence—10 or 20 years, but then it is over. For others, like myself, it is a life sentence. We may get some fleeting reprieve from pain medications and muscle relaxers for 4 to 6 hours when the meds first kick in. But unlike morphine, which separates the patient from the pain like an invisible shield, my pain "killers" merely dull the pain: It never totally goes away.

It has been 7 years since my accident, and my life has been altered irrevocably. I walk with a cane because of weakness in my knees and my diminished sense of balance. In 7 years, I have attended the cinema only twice because I cannot sit in one position for very long before my muscles knot up and cause pain. If I adjust my posture to find a comfortable position, I annoy fellow spectators, so it's best that I don't go to the cinema or other public events. I especially fear rock concerts because the audiences can be unpredictable and have even stampeded on occasion.

My occasional lower-back back pain began in college when I took stage combat and classes in Asian forms of self-defense. I moved wrong just enough to do some unknown thing to my spine; thereafter, the pain flared up two or three times a year and prevented me from standing up and moving about in comfort. My back pain was exacerbated by my accident 20 years later.

My *chronic* pain began with the accident. I was walking across the street inside the marked crosswalk when I was hit by a car speeding in the school zone. As I watched in slow motion, the front bumper got closer, struck my left knee and thigh, and sent me flying across the intersection. As I landed on my right side, the insides of my knees banged together.

The primary pain at the base of my spine is intense enough to make the insides of my teeth hurt. My earlier lower-back pain has now spread to include my midback and other apparently unrelated areas of my body. And now the pain is constant. Doctors have tried to find the causes of my various pains to no avail. According to the x-rays, CT scans, MRIs, and EMGs, nothing was broken—and yet, I am in constant pain.

Not even in sleep do I get relief: the pain prevents me from getting as much sleep as I need, and what sleep I do get does not make me feel rested. Getting to sleep has become difficult, and when I awaken, I still feel fatigued and sore. Of course, I can take antihistamines or sleeping pills, but I don't want to become even more dependent on meds to do something that I should be able to do on my own. Besides, sleep medications make me feel hung over; compounded by my general lack of rest, such drugs merely increase my feeling of perpetual fatigue.

When I'm awake, my general level of exhaustion feeds the pain and increases its intensity and duration—or my perception of it, at any rate. My best sleep comes from daytime naps. Sleep comes on quickly. I seem to sleep deeply, even if not for very long, because when I awaken, I usually feel more alert and rested and less drained and anxious.

New pains that have sprung up seem more neurological than muscular. Last year, I developed intense pains in my left elbow (a form of tennis elbow?). At the end of the summer, I had neurosurgery, and for a while, the procedure seemed successful; I felt better. Earlier this year, however, I developed corresponding pains on my right side, radiating from my elbow down into my forearm and up my arm to just short of my shoulder. These shooting pains are exacerbated when I write (which I do a great deal, as both a writer and a teacher). But equally disturbing are the dead hands. I need not do anything, or have my hands in any particular position, for my hands to fall asleep: They tingle—if that—and are otherwise numb and useless. Recently, regaining sensation in my hands has taken longer, and now I must vigorously massage feeling back into them.

These new pains are not restricted to my arms and hands. Of late, I can be sitting reading or writing, when sharp pains start shooting up and down my legs, and my feet tingle or feel numb, to the point that I cannot immediately stand on them.

Describing Pain

How do we describe something for which there are no precise words? It is extremely difficult because we must depend on similes and analogies to convey experiences and sensations that may correspond to something in the reader's own life.

I have finally arrived at a more accurate image of my "dead" hands: the sensation is like the numbness I experience under Novocaine, when my lips feel huge and rubbery—not really mine. In the same way, my hands are mine—but they're not. They're incapable of doing anything I want them to do. I can't control anything I feel.

I simply want this to stop. I can't stand being out of control. I'm so tired of being tired and I'm sore from being sore. I'm tired of being in pain. I'm pained from being in pain. I feel as though I'm reaching a threshold. Even with mood enhancers to keep me from going off the deep end, I still have images of opening my wrists in a sustained, tight-focus movie shot. I don't see the cutting, but I know it's done with a Swiss army knife. Either there is no sound or the soundtrack has been turned off. All is silent, calm.

The pain in my elbows is like a spike, a sharpness that penetrates. I can feel it enter and exit. Lately, it has felt even finer than the spike. Today, it's more like a steel knitting needle with a slender point that gradually becomes thicker and more spikelike.

This sharp sense of vibrating penetration conjures up a portrait of Saint Sebastian, pierced with arrows: this is how I feel. But Sebastian died. His physical pain ceased; his torture ended at least. In my imagination, my arrows are electrified. They automatically twist and thrust in and out, doubly reminding me that they're in deep and that I am alive. But is this living?

Being in Pain

What is pain? Many illnesses result in pain—so is pain an illness?

If true, then I am ill because of pain. And what of these "peripheral" pains/illnesses I'm experiencing in my arms and hands and legs and feet? Do they stem only from the accident? If so, why have they only recently manifested themselves? One thing is clear: whatever the cause, my pain is real—so say my doctors.

Being in pain is to be constantly reminded that you are alive and trapped in your body. You feel less than generous toward the medical establishment, who can grant a prescription for drugs that bring temporary relief—or withhold medication and force you to beg. This same establishment neither sanctions suicide nor gives sufficient medication to deaden feeling in your body.

With sex, the body senses are heightened, ultimately to climax and release; but with pain, there is no release. The body is continuously in a high state of awareness—always tense, always on red alert. Pain is a constant, sometimes like low-grade fever and sometimes like burning flares—so intense you want to flay yourself just to get out of your body. Your muscles vibrate as if touching a live electrical socket. Even the inside of your head vibrates, causing changes in your vision. Simultaneously, you're detoxing so that you can maintain the effects of the medication. You find that you're taking more drugs with less relief because you've developed a tolerance—or worse, you discover you've run out before you're due for a renewal. The pains persist. They're never passive, but if you're lucky, the throbbing is at least dulled. When I'm moving, exercising, or otherwise distracted, my pain diminishes largely because I'm less aware of it: my consciousness is aimed elsewhere at specific tasks.

And as other ailments surface that need to be controlled, you get sucked ever deeper into your body, whose purpose is to carry the brain around and allow it to be in charge. But the brain cannot function properly. Its efficiency is short-circuited by the scraping sensation vibrating in the middle of your muscles or the center of your bones. Imagine running a knife edge across a dry, meatless, marrowless bone. That is what pain feels like. Pain decreases creativity and intellectual ability. It keeps you from giving everything to a task or a relationship.

The pain in my back is often unnaturally warm and pulsing. Frequently, it is a sharp, shooting pain, and sometimes it throbs, but not always. Sometimes I get a jabbing, stinging pain with each pulse.

And sometimes when the pain moves from my lumbar region up to the lower thoracic part of my back, a sharp pain shoots up my back like quicksilver, first starting in what feels like the center of the base of my spinal column (as if that could be) and then stabbing deeply in the surrounding muscles. When I recover enough so that I can move, my motion is restricted because if I move just wrong—even slightly—it can start again. So there is tension on two fronts: fear of moving incorrectly and anxiety about the pain that will result.

Identifying a "wrong" move in advance is difficult. I've thrown out my back while taking a shower or drying myself off, putting on my shoes or tying them or putting on my pants, and putting an arm through a shirt sleeve. There seems to be no singular, predictable action that regularly aggravates the pain.

Besides the weakness and soreness of my back, a noticeable consequence of my arm pains is the weakness in my right hand. I notice it when I shake hands (this is an embarrassment since I believe I once had a decent handshake) or open bottles or jars or lift books, even something as light as *The Dream of the Red Chamber*. My arm tires easily and pain mixes with fatigue when I write for too long, for instance, on a chalkboard. My hand and arm feel very heavy, even when I write in bed with the notebook propped against my knees.

I don't reflect on being in pain all the time. Like so many other things that one thinks about, I contemplate it during lulls, more often after the fact than during. When you're in pain, you're too occupied dealing with it—trying to reduce it or get rid of it—to have time to think about it. When I'm in the midst of an episode, engaging in an intellectual dialogue either with my rational self or with my pain (personified) generally doesn't work because I'm functioning on an emotional, not an intellectual, level.

Pain distorts one's perception of reality and makes living—or wanting to live—difficult. Whether I'm actively in pain or not, there's the dread of *being* in pain. This tempers how I feel about life and whether I want to continue living. When I think about living, I don't have pleasant images or feelings. Instead I picture the persistent vibrating pain moving up and down my spine or my arms. Or think about severing my wrists—although this wouldn't even be my preferred method of suicide and I have no memory of pain, of actually slashing the skin or the veins and arteries. But the *effect*! The life running out. Lying in a tub of warm water to keep the veins open, as did the Latin philosopher, or in a cold, empty tub watching the blood streak its way toward the drain—and down. But in a filled tub, water dilutes my life as I dwindle toward the shell that I've felt I've been for so long. It's like a vision becoming real.

Now, that Nothing has been replaced with pain. It has supplanted the Nothing that preexisted. But now I don't feel as vacant because the void has been filled by pain or its anticipation.

Being in Constant Pain

Being in pain has become a normal, transient, yet steady state—a constant. I cannot remember what being without pain is like. I can remember activities I used to be able to perform without pain, but not the experience of being pain-free. Not only is this frustrating; it is depressing to have but a vague sense, only through memories.

I've come to accept chronic pain as part of my existence. I think—I hope—I've gotten beyond the place of blaming anyone, especially the doctors who cannot diagnose the specific cause of the pain. I simply accept it as part of the landscape in which I exist and cope as best I can.

The most I hope for is that medication will dull the pain so that I can function without pulling out my hair. I can only hope to be distracted long enough to be able to work. For the 7 years I've been living with it, the most I can expect is to manage the pain, to make this existence bearable, which means masking the pain, since it won't go away.

I have talked about the effect of these various pains on the way I lead my life, about how I limit what I do. Actually, knowing when to stop a movement, or not to begin it at all, is simple: it is predicated on whether the movement causes pain, or increases it, or causes anxiety—or is even necessary at all. For example, I can walk if I can stand upright and my knees don't feel like they're going to buckle or if shooting pains don't run through them. Since I have found a walking partner and begun physical therapy, I seem to be able to walk better: more quickly, more easily, and with greater endurance.

I think I have come simply to accept that the pain's here and it is unlikely to go away. I try to accept it as part of my being right now, because I really have only two choices: to endure it or die. Thus far, I've chosen to exist, but sometimes just barely. Recently, I went to my first movie in 6 years just to see if I could handle it. And I did, although uncomfortably.

Since I'm usually in some state of pain, what do I often think about? Well, death, of course, but I have ever since I was a youngster. But now, thinking about death seems justified: I have more of a reason to want to die because it's a sure solution.

Although I don't feel as depressed as I did when I first began therapy many years ago, I do still have images of slashing my wrists, or of "waking up dead," although not by my hand, of just ceasing to be. If I died, then I'd be out of pain, because for pain to exist, there must be a host, and if the host is dead, there is no place for the pain to inhabit, so it would have to disappear. Dissipate. But I really don't feel depressed. So says logic. But I do feel other sensations like anger and frustration.

However, when I compare my pain with that of those whom I have taken care of, whose pain seemed truly unbearable, my pain seems so insignificant: Compared to them, what do I have to complain about? Shouldn't I be grateful for what I have? For simply being alive? Perhaps I should—and yet I want so very much *not to be*, to be unconscious forever, to be out of pain. To be gone. This is what I wish for. At a certain level, consciousness *means* pain (being in pain); that's the human condition. As I prepare to fall asleep, I fantasize that I can exhale totally and simply cease to be. Simply empty myself. I'd merely become the physical Emptiness that I've felt for so long.

What is it like emotionally and psychologically to have been in pain for so long? The effect is wearing, draining. I have little or no energy, and this makes me less stable, less predictable. At work I'm more testy than perhaps I used to be. I do try to keep my emotions tethered, but I am still likely to fly off the handle—or so it feels.

I've been in pain for so long I've forgotten what it's like not to be in pain. I can only remember actions I was once able to perform that required movement (just as I once unthinkingly accepted that I could move easily and freely through stage space). So I must have been sufficiently free of pain to perform these actions.

This is disheartening, especially since the future holds no promise of the pain abating and my free, easy movement being restored. Perhaps what adds to the pain in the present is the lack of hope of ever being pain-free. Life has become painful even if I'm in no pain at the moment simply because of the mere anticipation of pain; so I hurt doubly, from the anticipation of the pain (my muscles tense up) and from the pain itself.

Then there's the resentment from having missed so many events simply because either I hadn't the energy to attend events or if I had made plans, I was in too much pain to follow through.

Emotional and Psychological Aspects

So what do I get out of all this? Is this a way of getting attention? Is this an excuse to see doctors? If so, why? To feel special? Do I really need such attention? Is my life so desperate?

Or possibly I need medications to alter my perception of life. (This is how at least one of my doctors perceives my "need" for meds—and makes me feel guilty for seeking relief in this way.) There may be some truth to this, at least according to my internist. I could always resort to more "natural" kinds of consciousness-altering substances, which are not always available, but by getting meds from the doctor, I still function within societal boundaries: the meds I take are prescribed, and hence, legal. And I get to alter my consciousness, although this is not my intention in taking such meds. The problem is, I don't feel substantially different from the way I did before I began taking these meds, except that the pains don't bother me as much as when I'm not on medication.

I don't think the meds mask my feelings—or at least to the degree that I'm incapable of "feeling" anything. Although my mind is strong, I have not been able to mask the feelings. But even if I could, I wouldn't, because this would prevent me from feeling the full intensity of the emotional pain: the sadness, the depression. And this, too, reminds me that I'm alive.

But I wonder about what I feel. And as I do, I realize that I'm confused about what I feel because I've had to numb myself or I've become so inattentive—I try not to ignore what goes on with me that isn't directly connected to my pain, because pain has become so overwhelming. And yet, here I've been asked to write about the pain in my life—or should I say, my life of pain—and this requires that I be conscious and attentive both to the pain and to the rest of my existence. In truth, both are a jumble—I'm not certain what I think, what I feel physically aside from pain, or what I feel emotionally.

I don't think ahead any more, for the most part because the future holds only more of the same: the anticipation of pain and the pain itself. This isn't to say that I live totally in the realm of memory, but memory has gained increasing import. I don't just wax nostalgic; I reconsider events from the past with fresh eyes (eyes perhaps rose-tinted by idealistic memory). I now consider which memories are worth remembering—and why. What have they to offer? Do they illuminate?

I began seeing a psychiatrist to try to answer the question my internist posed: "What do you get out of all this?" What *do* I get out of all this? This isn't just a question, it reflects an attitude, and it's just the somewhat antagonistic attitude that Job's "friends" maintained, the attitude that my rheumatologist conveyed that helped me decide not to see him anymore.

What I don't need (besides the physical pains) is to have to deal with someone else's "attitude" or feel guilty and anxious about something I don't seem to be able to do anything about. I have begun going to a pain clinic. I have begun exercising more regularly. I see that I *can* have some say and *can* take a more active role in dealing with the symptoms even if no one else can determine what's wrong with me. But what I don't need is psychobabble on top of trying to cope with pain. Sometimes I feel too fragmented, too kaleidoscopic; each image is complete, albeit askew. Each image is just "off" enough to distort what is real.

Being in Control

Being able to discern what is real is important to my sense of control, so I *must* assert command over as much as I can. I have been a control freak for years; I *must* be in command of all situations and conditions I'm in. Pain robs me of that control. Why exactly I feel that I must have such control is not totally clear. I suspect that situations and conditions in the past were not under my control and I try to compensate.

However, everything I do is predicated on how I feel at any given moment: my various body parts or my head or the two in tandem. This means that I can't always plan activities, or I can plan events but there is no guarantee that I'll actually be able to participate in them. Spontaneity is no longer part of my experience. My life has become less predictable, more out of control—and if anything distresses me, it is the loss of control over my life. I don't like that. I don't like being out of control.

Another manifestation of not being in control is my not knowing what I'm experiencing. On occasion, I feel surges of power propelling me through space, and I feel analogous urges to do "I don't know what" because I feel so crazy from the various pains. I get the crazy impulse to become extremely violent and smash something or someone's face—to hurt someone! Just as I feel that I have this desire to control my becoming dead. I have this desire to self-destruct, to end the pain. But in both cases, I've not acted.

The purpose of retaining control is to have some say while one is alive, and this long episode in pain has forced me to reevaluate whether staying alive is really worth enduring. In fairness to life, however, I have arrived at some grounds for considering living preferable. One reason for not committing suicide is that I am too fearful of many things in this world, especially the pain one would experience doing the deed, even though it could be the last pain I'd feel. And anyway, should I give the satisfaction to the creeps who would applaud such an act?

The rationale that others give for not committing suicide is that it would hurt them. The implicit message is that suicide is a selfish act. But I have difficulty accepting this reason because I cannot fathom how my presence or absence would make a bit of difference. Life will go on just as it always has. The presence of others makes sense to me because they have things to contribute. But one reason I have used to keep myself alive is the sense of incredulity of not being around to know what might be just around the corner: curiosity. To want to know. This is best manifested in a basic mime image of this sense.

Being in constant pain, then, is often like having my life on hold. I don' t know what I can do, what to do, or when I can do it. This is probably the most irritating part of my situation.

Diverse Observations

I suspect that what or who I am is decided by what kind of pain, and how much pain, I'm in. I can no longer remember a time when I wasn't in pain. The last 7 years have pretty much become fused and fuzzy and have overwhelmed any memories of my life before this intense, chronic pain that has changed my life to an existence. I can recall only colorless memories of what I've done in the past, such as traveling, living, and studying abroad, but I can't remember what they felt like because pain filters and interferes with even my memories. I can't call up memories of *physical* activities. For instance, I can recall going to the Comédie Française, but I can't remember actually sitting through *Le Bourgeois Gentilhomme* for however long it lasts and recalling how it felt to be so caught up in the play that I'd forget myself, because if I try, all I can call up is how painful it would be now to even go to such an event. (I angered my neighboring spectators at the last play I saw because I couldn't sit still.)

And since I've been in pain for so long, I've lost any idea of what it means to be or feel normal, namely, without pain. Because of this, when my friends talk about mundane things in their lives that I used to be able to partake in, such as a sex life, I feel as though I were an alien and that they're talking about something that exists only as a vague memory. To put it another way, it's like listening to a language that I can't participate in because I no longer have the common referents. Perhaps a kind of alienation has set in, but an estrangement different from that which results from living in these post-existential times.

The other observation that is probably a corollary to the first is that I've come to identify with the pain. The pain and I have become inseparable: it's hard to know where I leave off and the pain begins. And it's for this reason that how much of who I really am now is shaped and masked by pain, and so the duration and intensity of pain can determine what or who emerges to deal with life, which, for the most part, has become a pain—pained life.

I consider what being in pain is like by looking at how it has affected the way I now live my life. Most obviously, my life is more sedentary. But how much of this is because of pain and how much is due to aging, I'm not certain. No doubt, it's a combination of both. I've pretty much retreated within my apartment to the sanctuary of my books and music.

Since I've been depressed for so long—long before I hurt myself—I can no longer tell if I'm this way because of the constant pain or because of other factors. What I do suspect, however, is that I'm more irritable because of the pain. I'm probably more likely to fly off the handle, especially when dealing with 150 adolescents a day.

If I do reflect on these pains, which I'm bound to do, and if I do feel depressed, perhaps it is because I think of the things I can no longer do.

I cannot

- Move freely, easily.
- Sit still for long periods, which means I can't go to plays, movies, or concerts.
- Give a good handshake because my right hand and arm hurt and have become weakened. This embarrasses me.
- Lift even moderately light objects, like books, without feeling either weakness or shooting pain up and down my right arm.
- Write by hand for long stretches because my hand cramps up.
- Control (well, it's becoming increasingly more difficult) these destructive images and urges.
- Control my moods.
- Make plans to do things or go places because everything is subject to change, depending on how I feel at the appointed time. (How many activities have I had to cancel because I didn't feel well enough?)
- Become involved in a relationship even if I were interested in one because even the thought of having to bottle up negative feelings to spare the other person makes me feel as though I might explode.
- Even think about having a sex life because my sex drive is so minimal, erratic, or nonexistent. In truth, this is just as well, because it's one less thing to have to deal with.

I cannot

- Keep up with my paperwork from my job.
- Work on my dissertation and finish the bloody degree.
- Not think about or feel pain. Even if I do relaxation exercises, I'm still, at some level, aware of how much I hurt. Equally annoying as the sharp, stabbing, shooting pains are the persistent, dull chest pains that have developed and are now simply there, especially those that band around to my back. But I am aware at all times of these pains, even when the interior work that I'm doing to alleviate pain is working.
- Not be conscious or aware of my body even when my attention should be focused elsewhere, like on my mind. The pain makes me want to cut off that part of my body that hurts—or take off my body, as one does an uncomfortable shirt.
- Control my life. I can't be spontaneous. I am subject to doing whatever the pain permits me to do.
- Be drugged up as much as I want. The drugs don't make the pains go away; they don't (according to my internist) make me addicted to them or give me a buzz. They only make the pain tolerable by dulling it.

Now, sharp pains are shooting through both my arms. My head aches, but it can't be because of my blood pressure, which is usually within tolerable limits. (It's high when I awake, but it usually drops to normal levels as the day progresses.) My headaches are one of two types unless they combine: a band around my head or a pressing of the sides of my head just above my ears.

CRITICAL-THINKING ACTIVITIES

1. Describe the elements of Greg Lum's chronic pain that make his experience seem like a life sentence—a prisoner of pain. How do his descriptions assist the practitioner in diagnosing and helping the writer manage his constant pain?

2. How have the author's accident and its sequelae affected the quality of his life? Explain in detail.

3. How would you assist the writer in resolving his sleep disturbance? Create a collaborative model of care, taking into account the potential problems of the interaction of pain analgesics and sleep medication and Lum's need for a clear mind in order to teach.

4. Lum compares certain health-care providers with the friends of Job (the biblical hero who was afflicted with dire misfortunes and whose friends essentially blamed him for those afflictions). Compare and contrast Job's friends with the providers in this narrative and discuss the implications of their behavior and actions.

5. Lum asks, "What is pain? Many illnesses result in pain—so is pain an illness?" Elaborate on this conjecture and discuss its implications.

6. What is your understanding of the doctor's question, "What is this pain keeping you from doing?" Could this question in any way stigmatize the sufferer? How? What do you suggest as a helpful way of assisting Lum?

7. Lum states that he wonders if he sounds depressed, crazy, or suicidal and then adds, "I'm all three." How could this be so? What exactly has occurred that has led to these afflictions?

8. Lum describes a solitary life devoid of interests and activities that he enjoys and that are necessary for his personal fulfillment. What would you say or do if he told you this? Explain your answer, keeping in mind the severity of his situation.

9. How might health-care professionals overcome their fear and dismay of individuals who have chronic, debilitating, undiagnosed pain? Discuss in detail.

10. Describe the ways in which the voice and style of writing of this author enable the health-care professional student to understand the vicious cycle of pain, anger, fear, and hopelessness inherent in the lives of those who suffer with chronic pain.

11. Write a paper in which you research the current practice or models of care for those who suffer with debilitating, chronic pain from which there seems no hope for remission.

David Gordon

David Gordon is a writer now living in the Boston area, where some years earlier he completed an MA in creative writing. He is the author of several nonfiction books and is currently attempting to market a screenplay and complete a novel about near-death experiences. Though he is also working on a PhD in English, his ambition is to live in a small house by the ocean, where he can become light again.

Here Gordon meticulously records the horrifying and mystifying events of a near-death experience and his hospitalization and surgery for a hemorrhage of unknown origin. He examines the attitudes and behaviors that he believes contributed to his near demise and also interfered, and still interfere, with his recovery.

CHAPTER 9

Reconceptions

by David Gordon

*E*ach January 19th, at about eight o'clock in the evening, I perform a combined memorial service and birthday celebration. I light a candle that I keep on the top shelf of a small desk I've set up as a makeshift altar. Beside the candle are a large piece of obsidian, a few photographs of myself hang-gliding in France, and a small leather box. After I light the candle, I retrieve a microcassette from the box, which also contains a St. Christopher's medal, a Dr. Who pin, a smaller piece of obsidian, and a piece of cardboard shaped like a tombstone. I place the tape in my tape recorder and record the Jewish memorial prayer, then I reflect out loud on the events of the preceding year and my hopes for the coming one.

These past three years Hatsune, my girlfriend, has been part of this ceremony, as she was part of the events I commemorate. But I would perform the ceremony without her, too.

The memorial is for the parts of me that died at that hour, on that day in 1992, at Sisters of Mercy Hospital in Syracuse, New York. The cardboard tombstone acknowledges the service that those dead parts rendered to me; the medal symbolizes the hospital's Catholicism; the pin, my visit to another reality; the obsidian, what I saw while I was there. The celebration is for the parts of me that were born a few minutes later (the first year, Hatsune and I ate birthday cake, and I made a wish and blew out one candle), and the photographs are part of the hoped-for future.

Historically, my actual birthday (which comes 3 weeks later) has been an important time for me, a day on which significant things have tended to happen, a day during which I have evaluated my past and prepared for my future. Although I still acknowledge that day, it doesn't mean as much to me anymore. January 19, the anniversary of the day I died, more *or* less, and came back, more *and* less, has pretty much replaced it.

Near Dead

On that evening in 1992 I suffered what I guess would be called a vascular accident, in my case an accident of birth waiting to happen for nearly 41 years.

Its initial warning sign was moderate gastrointestinal bleeding, perhaps a pint lost per day, which on the second day brought me into the emergency room of Sisters'

Hospital. I expected to have a few tests and go home (this was on a crisp Saturday afternoon) but allowed them to admit me when the emergency room doctor said that although they couldn't test me till Monday, I'd better stay because, as he put it, "Sometimes these things really let loose. You may not be able to get back here in time."

The tentative diagnosis was lower bowel ulcers induced by a month on Motrin for a shoulder ailment, a course of medication I'd just completed. In the backs of their minds the Sisters' Hospital doctors may also have been thinking "cancer," but I didn't even think about that until much later. At first I was merely irritated at the inconvenience, the time I would miss from work, and the potential cost—my insurance is not the best. I became genuinely concerned only when the gastroenterologist they assigned to me said she didn't *think* she'd have to transfuse, but she was ordering blood of my type, just in case. She also said she didn't think they'd have to operate. Until that moment it had not even occurred to me that they might transfuse, or operate, or that there was anything seriously wrong. Except for a little weakness, I felt fine.

I remained at Sisters' all of Saturday and Sunday, drinking clear liquids and sucking in IV fluids. By Sunday night the bleeding had stopped and they wanted to give me a strong laxative to "clean me out" so they could "scope" me the following morning. Their hope, and by then mine, was that they would find large surface ulcers, would inject them with something to stop the bleeding, and would send me home in a couple of days with medications and a bland diet. I resisted the laxative—it seemed a bad idea to stir up bleeding tissues—but the doctor and nurses insisted that short of exploratory surgery, theirs was the only way to find out what was wrong. Reluctantly, I agreed.

Once the cathartic had started to do its work, I produced a toilet bowl filled, it seemed to me, with blood. The nurse—who couldn't have been more than 20 and who, I later learned, had failed the examination that would have promoted her from LPN to RN—said I'd expelled about 300 cc. She flushed away the evidence, then left to consult with a more senior nurse. When she returned about 15 minutes later, she told me they'd called the gastroenterologist. The doctor had said this was just old blood, was expected, and merely indicated that the medicine was "doing what it was supposed to do." I was not reassured, but I accepted this diagnosis; I didn't feel as if I had much choice. Now, in retrospect, I realize I could probably have insisted on waiting a few more days before they had administered the medication in the first place, and I should certainly have insisted on seeing a doctor right then. But I wanted to believe them. I wanted to believe that everything would be just fine if I left things in their hands.

About an hour later, on my way back from my fourth trip to the bathroom, I blacked out before I could reach the nurse's call button. I remember weakly crying for help and collapsing to my knees, fearing that my call would go unheard.

This fear was not groundless. A hospital is never quiet. At that time, there were two geriatric patients around the corner who moaned or cried out periodically throughout most of the day and fairly late into the night. One moaned roughly every 30 seconds. When the moaner started, the other cried out "Help me!" about once a minute. There was also some kind of monitor nearby that would periodically make a beep followed by a chord of two or three beeps. This sound seemed to trigger the moans and the cries for help, much as a siren might excite the neighborhood dogs. Even with ear plugs, I had been able to hear these moans and cries.

"I'd rather be dead than end up like that," I had said to Hatsune earlier that day.

"You shouldn't say that!" she scolded. "God will hear!"

As I lost consciousness, I realized that my cries would sound no different from theirs, and I feared that, as with the boy who cried wolf, nobody would distinguish the real emergency from the false alarm, perhaps not even God.

The next thing I remember is two nurses crouching beside me as I lay on my back in a pool of blood. I had probably been out 10 or 15 minutes, and when they roused me, my blood pressure was quite low, 70 over 50 or thereabouts. I felt very cold.

The nurses put a sheet under me, got a couple of extra pairs of hands from the hallway, and together hoisted me onto the bed, where they began to infuse liquids. At first they thought they could stabilize me with fluids, but they were wrong, because I began to bleed again, heavily, a few minutes later. I could feel the blood pouring out of me, rolling up my backside, along my back. It was a welcome warmth, like peeing in a wet suit.

They started a transfusion, and that, too, seemed to help me at first, but again I started to bleed, this time pumping blood out faster than they could pump it back in. I kept telling them I was cold. They kept telling me, "You're not going to die, don't worry, you're not going to die." Then they attempted to start another unit of blood, but they couldn't find a vein—my blood pressure was so low (it eventually dropped to 50 over 0, effectively flat) that the veins in my arms had collapsed. They stopped telling me I was going to be all right and started calling for things *stat*.

At that point I realized that I *could* die. Until then, I had been curiously detached from my situation, had felt as if I were at home watching television and all this fuss was happening somewhere else, to someone else. But when I saw that the doctor and nurses were no longer in control, it became clear to me that I might have only a couple of minutes left to live.

I was completely unafraid. As the room began to fade out around me, I saw a series of charts that represented the course of my life, somewhat like the overlays of the human body's various systems one sees in anatomy texts. The chart on top represented my vocation; it dipped down in the bad times—the longest being my recent decade in industry—and up in the good times, when I had quit the business world and gone back to graduate school. Lower charts showed similar patterns in other aspects of my life: family, romantic relationships, others I no longer recall.

As I lost all bodily sensation, I felt a surge of regret not so much for the things I had done as for the things I had not done, either because I was following someone else's bidding or because I was cutting off my own desires, taking the apparently easier route. Then the regret passed and I felt as if the books had been balanced and closed on my life. Yet I didn't want to die. So I made a case, for myself and for God, if there is one, and if he was listening, to let me continue. I felt I understood how to live my life, finally, and I wanted a chance to complete it. Then the room and my body faded out and "I" went into another space entirely.

I am in a black, dimensionless room—that is what I see, although there is no particular "I" doing the seeing. All the walls and ceilings lean at angles that defeat normal rules of perspective, and the surfaces glint, as if they are made of chipped flint or obsidian. The effect is somewhat like that of moonlight on choppy seas: it is the reflection of light you see, not the waves themselves, and the reflections shift as the waters tumble.

I feel no anxiety, hear no sounds, have no memories, think no thoughts. I am unaware of the passage of time. I am more alone than I've ever been, but it doesn't bother me.

My memory of events that followed the near-death experience is less clear. Shortly after I regained consciousness, Hatsune arrived. She seemed calm, almost cheerful, as I told her briefly what had happened to me. Later, she said that the bed was soaked with red, and that the room smelled like a woman's period. She asked me if she could pray for me, and I said yes, but when she ended the prayer, "In Jesus' name, amen," I told her I did not believe in Jesus.

Next I remember being cleaned up and then lifted onto a gurney by four people, who carefully manipulated what had become an array of IV poles. While I waited for a room in the intensive care unit (ICU), I asked Hatsune to call my mother and my brother Richard, and I requested that Richard come to Syracuse if he could. Hatsune and the nurses all tried to keep me talking, keep me conscious, but this didn't seem to be a problem: I was back. As they wheeled me down to the ICU, I was very talkative, attempting to make small jokes. My focus was almost entirely outward, as if I were trying to make a good impression on the nurses and doctor. Perhaps I felt they would take better care of me if I did that—if I seemed to be a person, not just a patient.

The ICU nurses were all female, and they introduced themselves to me in turn. I no longer remember any of their names, though I have their observations in my chart. The overhead lights in the ICU seemed very bright, like the sodium lamps outside a shopping mall.

The gastroenterologist, who had also accompanied me down to the ICU, asked me to sign a permission form for an endoscopic examination, then she inserted a camera in my nostril, and worked it down into my stomach and beyond. I remember protesting that they had looked there already—this was the third time they had inserted something through my nose and down my throat, the first in the ER, the second just after I had "come to"—but the doctor insisted that there might be bleeding in the duodenum and this was the easiest way to find out. Gagging and choking as the tube went down, I thought of the drunk who drops his keys in the driveway but looks for them by the street light because the light is better there: they were looking where it was easy, not where the trouble was more likely to be found.

They inserted a catheter in my neck and worked it down the jugular vein. Then one of the nurses attempted to insert a urinary catheter, but she couldn't get the tube past my prostate gland. I remember screaming through the entire procedure; Hatsune said she could hear my screams from the waiting room down the hall. I refused to let them try again without giving me pain killers.

If there is a distinction between experiencing and remembering, it is lost on doctors. When the chief resident arrived, I repeated my request for pain killers; by this time my penis was on fire from the first catheterization attempt. He said pain was an important indicator of what was going on inside me and they needed to know when and where I hurt. He could apply a local pain killer to the tube, which would help with the pain of insertion; for the rest, he would give me something to relax me that would also erase my memory of the pain. I agreed to all this—again, I seemed to have no choice—but thought, "Great, I'll suffer but I won't remember it, and that's supposed to make it okay?"

In fact, however, in a way he was right. I remember the injection—it felt as if I were standing under a waterfall, pelted by rushing water—but I don't remember much of what happened for the remainder of the night or during the following day. Much later, the resident explained that they intentionally give surgical patients drugs that not only relax them but also erase short-term memory so that they will forget anything they hear or feel while they are under anesthesia. But is not remembering really the same as not feeling, not knowing, in the first place?

Early the next morning I apparently bled again and was again transfused. I don't remember. The ICU nurse who administered the blood wrote in my chart that I said I was afraid I would die, but I don't remember that conversation, either. According to the resident, he and I had a long discussion about my options and I agreed first to an angiogram and then to surgery, but that memory, too, has been erased. My only clear memories are of being roused repeatedly to sign various permission forms. The sensation was as if I were writing on water rather than paper, the characters of my name created as if by magic, the resulting signature of the last form I signed not unlike my nearly blind grandmother's unreadable scrawl. According to my chart, I also gave oral permission for them to remove sections of my small and large intestine, though I don't see how I could have—I was unconscious at the time. But again, I don't remember.

Later that morning they prepped me for major abdominal surgery. Beginning at noon, in a 4-hour operation, they opened me from breastbone to pubic bone, palpated my intestinal tract, and in their heavy-handed way removed everything they thought might be bleeding.

There were two possible sites for the bleeding: one a small pouch on my small intestine they had not expected to find and the other a possible arterial defect in the juncture between small and large intestine known as the cecum. The surgeon removed both, which also meant removing several feet of large and small intestine and the ileal-cecal valve that connects them. My brother Richard, a veterinary surgeon, later questioned the chief surgeon about his having performed such radical surgery. In the manner that turned out to be typically his, the surgeon explained, "There was a gallon of blood in there, and the angiogram said the bleeding was from the cecum. I'd have looked like a damn fool if I didn't get the bleeder and we had to go back in again the next day."

Immediately after surgery, the surgeon told me he was sure the bleeding had been from the cecum. A day later, after he received the pathologist's report, he reversed this diagnosis. There was nothing wrong with the intestines he'd removed. Only the small pouch had contained damaged blood vessels.

■

The room is some sort of cave, apparently manmade, possibly open to the outside, but dark except for reflections of light on the sharp edges of the side walls and the ceiling. The light comes from the center of the room where, as my consciousness moves forward, I see there is sketched, in lines of solid white light, like neon tubes or glowing pipe cleaners, a rough table and an approximation of a chair. Seated on the chair, its back to me, is a manboy, also drawn in white light.

The creature is not drawn in detail. I can see only a squared-off oval for a head and a loose collection of lines for the body and arms, as if it had been created by a child or by a cartoonist trying to draw like a child. It appears to be leaning on the table with one arm, its chin in its hand, and perhaps it—he, I may as well say he—is holding a pen in the other hand, resting it on the table as if poised in thought.

■

In the end it was not cancer or a bowel ulcer, as the gastroenterologist had earlier speculated, or an arterial defect, as the surgeon had believed during the operation, or any of the other ravages of age that the doctors at Sisters' Hospital had suspected, but an umbilical remnant, a small pouch known as Meckel's diverticulum, that had nearly finished me.

I left the hospital knowing only that what had caused me to bleed could not recur and that it was a rare condition—though some 2 percent of the population is born with it, according to the surgeon, in only "one in a thousand, in ten thousand" cases does it sit quiescently well beyond childhood, an organic bomb waiting for the right trigger to set it off. For a while, this information was enough; I had to get on with life. But as I began to recover, I wanted to know more, maybe even to write about this condition so as to alert other physicians and nurses to its possibility and perhaps save others from unnecessarily radical surgery.

I began by asking my brother Richard to look into the subject. "Let me explain what I understand about this thing," Rick wrote. "As a fetus, you need four things: oxygenated blood to flow into your arteries, deoxygenated blood to drain out of your veins to get reoxygenated, a way to eliminate liquid waste, and a way to get rid of solid waste. The umbilical cord provides ways to do all of these."

He then explained that at each of the umbilical cord attachments, the fetus has special structures designed to circumvent the still-developing organs of the fetus. They are known as the ductus arteriosus, which bypasses the lungs; the urachus, which bypasses the urinary tract; and the vitelline stalk, which bypasses the colon. All of these structures are supposed to close off completely at birth so that the fetus's own mechanisms for oxygenating blood and eliminating waste can take over. Normally, they are then absorbed completely into the newborn's body.

"If the vitelline stalk doesn't close," my brother wrote, "the animal may have a complete tube which carries feces from the intestine to the belly button, or only a remnant of the duct called Meckel's diverticulum. The open ductus arteriosus, open urachus, and Meckel's diverticulum all share one feature: they are caused by failure of a structure which was essential to the life of the fetus to completely close once birth takes place. What I did not know is that in people, at least, the Meckel's is lined by cells which produce acid just like the cells which line the stomach. What most likely happened in your case is that the Motrin stimulated acid production in both your stomach and in your diverticulum. For natural reasons or perhaps because you took antacids, the stomach was able to handle the added acid production, but the diverticulum was not. The acid ate through a blood vessel in the diverticulum and caused your bleeding."

It is seldom good to be a medical anomaly.

------- ■ -------

My sense is that this creature is me, the me I was born with, the me I would die with, my essential Self; that it is waiting; and that it can continue to wait indefinitely. I do not wonder what will happen next. I am content to just wait there, being him and watching him at the same time.

Then my consciousness zooms suddenly forward, and as it does, the figure at the table turns his head toward me so that I can see the outline of his face, the sharp angle of his chin, his nose pointed and elongated in profile. He seems almost to be smiling.

A moment later I am back in my hospital bed, bathed in my own blood, another person's blood flowing into my left arm from two IV needles and a pair of plastic bags. A nurse is reading off my blood pressure: "70 over 30." "80 over 50." "90 over 60." The doctor's narrow face looms over me, a nervous smile. "There, that's better," she says, flushed and sweaty. "Isn't that better?"

Time

My first experience of time as a continuum occurred when I was about 10 years old. Before that, I think time was invisible to me.

I was riding my bike past Johnny Sybulski's house and I stopped, suddenly, for no particular reason. I looked at the simple brick facade, the white trim, the unkempt bushes, and I became aware of myself looking. I thought, "This is just one second in my life, and I'll never remember it again." But that moment is one of my more vivid memories from childhood. It marked the beginning of my sense of myself as mortal.

Both of my grandfathers had died that year. In each case I had seen them nearing death in the hospital some weeks before and had seen their dead bodies in the funeral home. Perhaps that's why I noticed that moment, or perhaps 10 is when most boys begin to understand time and death; I don't know. What I do know is that from that point on, time had a kind of linearity it had not had before, and this linearity soon became part of my background understanding of the cosmos. As I got older, time became invisible again, but differently than it had before.

Dr. Stephen L. Thaler, a physicist who has modeled near-death and death itself on a neural network, believes that as neurons die, the surrounding neurons experience the loss of their compatriots as life events. Somewhat like dreams or hallucinations, the death visions created by dying neurons are as real to the dying person as anything else he or she has ever experienced. Thaler hypothesizes that this process continues until death is complete, and that "for all intents, the dying individual may experience forever, through the cascading death of nearly 100 billion brain cells (and an unfathomable number of interconnections) within an instant, resulting in a torrent of experience tantamount to eternity. It is as if life is going on for the trauma victim. However, the time-line at death has only a moment's projection on the timeline we call 'real.'"*

According to the doctor and the nurses who resuscitated me, my near-death experience must have lasted no more than a minute or two. They said I was talking to them all the while they were attempting to transfuse me, and that even during the blackout period I had continually crossed my hands over my chest, perhaps in an effort to warm myself. (Like Snowden in *Catch-22*, I was cold, so cold). They seemed surprised when I told them I'd had a near-death experience. Busy with trying to keep me alive, they hadn't noticed I'd left the room.

During that minute or two of *their* time, however, my time seemed infinite, my experience of being alive at once the most intense and the simplest of my recollected existence. In near-death, time does more than slow down, as it might during a more routine emergency. It changes altogether, collapses into a singularity and then spans out again, altered, like light refracted by a prism.

After surgery, time moved in a jerky fashion. No longer stopped dead, as it had been during the near-death experience, time nevertheless stretched out almost endlessly. Days went on forever, much as they had when I was a child, and the 2 weeks I spent at Sisters' Hospital seemed—still seem, today—to contain the experience of years.

Those days are by far the longest of my existence, but this way of experiencing time continued for several months. Later, when I began to circulate among the ordinary living again, I felt as if decades had passed. It was as though I had been rewarded for my troubles with an elongated sense of time. This seemed good. But it was also as if I were a modern incarnation of Rip Van Winkle, returning to a time and place that had moved on without me, a people among whom I could walk but with whom I no longer belonged. I could not talk about the things I had once cared about, could not easily pick up any of the activities I left behind. I had been away too long and had forgotten my old ways.

Like before, time had become visible.

Now I think about time a good deal more than I used to, especially during the gaps between ending one thing and beginning another, the "waiting for a bus" times: waiting for someone to pick up the phone as it rings, waiting for a television commercial to end, waiting for my computer to save a file so I can get back to work. Those times. I think about the minute or two I was over there, on the "other side," or if not *there*, then very close to it, and of the similarities and differences between that minute or two and those others. (Waiting for a bus and waiting to die are both, after all, waiting, though in the for-

*Steven L. Thaler, "Death of a Gedanken Creature," *Journal of Near-Death Studies*, 13(3):164, 1995.

mer very little seems to change, while during the latter, when life actually *was* on hold, everything did.) Then I think about other minutes that divide everything into before and after: the minute you find out your mate is having an affair, your boss tells you you're fired, your doctor tells you you have cancer, your car slides out of control. Or the other side of the equation: the minute a child is born, a lottery won, a love relationship consummated. These minutes, too, contain more life in them than an average month of ordinary and predictable experience, and I wonder why it is that instead of seeking out the moments when every drop of life, bitter or sweet, is hot and passionate, most of us gravitate toward those empty minutes, find comfort in those in-between times.

In the ensuing months since my near-death experience, time has once again started to become invisible, and as the years pass I suspect this process will continue. But as before, it will do so differently.

Reconception

The medical term for hauling someone back from the brink of death is *"resuscitation,"* the act of restoring consciousness, vigor, or life. This term is perhaps too arrogant in its attribution: both the mechanism by which one is revived and the factors that determine who lives and who dies are far from understood. A better term might be *"resurrection,"* the act of rising from the dead, which leaves the causal agent unstated—God, medicine, will to live, and luck are equal contenders. To one who has been there and back, however, neither term feels quite right. Coming back from a near-death experience feels less like resuscitation or resurrection, both of which imply a return to what was, than it does like rebirth, a second or new birth, a reincarnation.

But even rebirth does not precisely describe the moment of near-death itself.

I think it was the critic Kenneth Burke, speaking of Saint Augustine's *Confessions,* who said that autobiography puts a stop to the part of a life that has already happened, like ending a sentence with a period. A new life, like a new sentence, takes place from that point forward.

I believe that near-death, like autobiography, divides what was from what will be. To continue the analogy, the period at the end of my sentence—the end of my original life, the life my parents gave me—occurred when I lost conventional consciousness at about 8 P.M. on Sunday, January 19, 1992. A new life—the life I'm in now, a life I requested as the room grew dim around me—began a few minutes later. The near-death experience, therefore, was the white space that separates that old life, that previous sentence, and this one; not so much a rebirth as a repetition of the act of conception: a *reconception,* in all of its layered meanings.

The events that followed parallel the events that follow conventional conception:

■ *Regestation.* In the operating theater, as in infancy, I was connected to apparatuses that supplemented or circumvented built-in mechanisms for taking in fuel and oxygen and eliminating the byproducts of metabolism. Aping the original umbilical connection, one tube fed me oxygen, another nourishment, and another removed waste, bypassing built-in structures that could not yet do what they were meant to do. If the near-death experience was reconception, then it follows that the surgery and early part of recovery were regestation.

■ *Reinfancy.* To extend the analogy, as the tubes were gradually withdrawn, I gained limited independence from my postsurgical womb. Still frail and helpless, I entered a second infancy in which, like a newborn, my basic needs were attended to by others.

■ *Regrowth.* Then, during the long recovery, at first in my mother's care and later in Hatsune's, I started to progress from this second infancy to second adulthood, replaying many of the emotional relationships and conflicts I had gone through beginning 40 years before: needing my mother, struggling with my father first for her attention and then later for his respect.

At the same time, of course, I made efforts to resume my old life. But nothing seemed to work quite as it had. It was as if something sealed since my childhood, perhaps even since birth, had cracked open and was in me, roaming, growing, maturing on its own while a phantom of the old me performed a version of the life I'd lived before.

This process continues to this day. At times I still feel as if I am floating between two worlds, not quite who I seem to be either to others or to myself. With some physical limitations, I do most of the "normal" things I once did, but it doesn't always feel like it is I who am doing them, rather some trace of myself that is keeping things going until an unspecified integration takes place. So far, the process of catching up to my chronological age seems to be one I perform asymptotically; like Zeno's Achilles, I almost—but never quite—reach that final destination.

From what I've read and seen, many of those who experience near-death go through something like this. But an irony of my situation is that this cycle of death and rebirth was set in motion by a leftover from my original birth, a vestigial link between my mother and my embryonic self, as if I had never quite severed the connection between us. A further irony is that, much as a buried trauma from childhood can explode cataclysmically later in life and in the explosion's aftermath induce personality transformation, I seem, through this process of death, rebirth, and regrowth, to have healed many of my childhood wounds.

Tibetan Buddhists, if I understand them correctly, believe that we are built of three parts: a subtle spirit that precedes physical embodiment, an identity we acquire as we go through life, and a physical form. They believe that at the point of death, the link between spirit, identity, and physical form is severed. Only the spirit moves on.

My experience jibes with that view. During my near-death experience, the creature in what I have come to call the Waiting Room was all that was left of my consciousness. It was as if he was who I was when I first came into the world and what would have remained, if anything, had I died. I could see it only because, in the process of dying, I had left behind everything else. In my case, however, the separation between spirit, identity, and form was elastic, and like Humpty Dumpty in reverse, all the pieces gradually came back together, more and less. The me that exists now is some kind of amalgam.

I don't know how this will wind up. All I do know for sure is that although it bears an almost uncanny resemblance to the life I lived before, this life I am in now does not feel like a continuation. In ways both obvious and subtle, my life is no longer, as the Talking Heads once put it, "The same as it ever was. The same as it ever was. The same as it ever was."

THE MEMORY EFFECTS OF HEAVY PAIN MEDICATION

An unfortunate effect of tranquilizers and heavy pain medication is that although one is reasonably lucid at the time, what happens in the short term does not carry over to long-term memory. So my recollections, at least of the external events of the first week or more following my near-death experience, are spotty at best.

If reminded, I can recall certain visits, though not necessarily on what day they occurred. If reminded, I can also sometimes recall certain conversations, though often I cannot.

Examples: Although I knew my brother Richard had come all the way from Cleveland, until several weeks later, when Hatsune told me he'd been with me both the night after surgery and all of the following day, I'd thought he had stayed only a couple of hours. Hatsune reports that in the ICU I said, "Tell me a story, Rick," and he told us the story of *Goldilocks and the Three Bears*. Richard told me that Hatsune then related a Japanese story about the origins of dance. At present, I don't remember those details, though for some reason I remember a Jewish rabbi stopping by with a rose while I was still hooked to the oxygen cylinders, and I remember Richard putting classical music on in what must have been my room in intensive care, and I remember the face of the man who wheeled me from intensive care to my other room, though I no longer remember being wheeled to the room, or ever having been in intensive care.

Another unfortunate effect of the drugs is that they made it impossible for me to write, even to keep simple lists, and so the only records I have of what went on—beyond floating impressions like those I have just described—are the recollections of the friends and hospital staff who observed me.

I resent having lost those days. They are a gaping hole at the center of the most critical period of my life.

I have tried to recover them.

In the process of this recovery, I have scrutinized my chart, and I have talked to friends and family who have visited me and to several of the medical personnel. At some point it is likely that their memories will become mine, much as the images from my childhood that are anthologized in my family's folklore have blended with the memories of my actual experience.

THE MORNING AFTER

On the morning after my near-death experience, Hatsune waited at the hospital. She arrived 2 or 3 hours before I went into surgery and stayed until early evening, when I returned to the ICU. She said that when she entered the ICU, I was in the fetal position, clutching the bed rail in my sleep. She also told me that during those first few days, I seemed almost holy.

According to her diary, she and I talked briefly about who she had called and who she had not, whether my insurance company and my employers had been told, and whether my car would be safe in the hospital lot. Then she went to my apartment to turn off my computer and pick up some of my things.

By the time she returned, my brother Richard had arrived. "I can't do much talking, but I can do listening," I apparently told him when he first arrived.

Rick wrote of his first impressions of me.

"You looked terrible, but in a reversible sort of way," he said, "not like the doomed people around you. You were pale, and your face looked fat or bloated. There were various drips going into you through various catheters. One catheter was in your jugular vein (left) and this was a triple lumen type which had running into it fluids and a separate bag of morphine. Blood was going into a different catheter, and your left hand had an arterial catheter in it which hooked up to an arterial blood pressure monitor. In addition to these you had an ECG hooked up, and a urinary catheter. There was a nasogastric tube in your nose, and a separate tube delivering oxygen to your nostrils.

"Your mouth looked dry to the point of being painful. I saw some Q-Tip-like swabs, and asked if I could moisten your mouth with these. The nurse said I could, and also that I could attempt to wake you.

"When I called your name, you immediately snapped open your eyes. I cannot really explain how odd this was, but your eyes would literally snap open and be as widely opened as your eyelids would stretch, so that white showed all the way around your iris. The best way I can explain it is that your eyes looked as if you were in complete terror.

"Initially I just said 'Hi,' and who I was. You could answer in two or three words at a time, after which your eyes would half close, you would pause, and then say a few more words. You knew who I was, and you said thanks for coming in to see you. If any period of time lapsed without me saying something your eyes would close again, only to snap open in that terrified manner every time I would start a new sentence. A typical conversation at this point might be:

RICK: The doctor (*at this point your eyes snap open*) said he thought everything went well. He is sure he got the source of the bleeding.

DAVID: (*eyes wide open*) Where was the (*eyes half closed, 30-second pause*) blood coming from?

RICK: He thinks it was from the cecum, but he took out the diverticulum as well.

DAVID: (*eyes still open as long as there was not a significant time lapse*) After I can think straight (*pause*) can you explain this to me?

"I think you get the idea. The best way I can explain it is that you were fully competent mentally for extremely brief periods of time, and that you were even able to think in abstract terms such as referring to the future, but that such periods of cognizance were extremely laborious, and were interspersed by long periods in which all you could do was stop thinking. I do not think you were sleeping, I just think your brain was in neutral. The oddest thing was the way your eyes reflected something which I cannot understand, but perhaps you do."

PAIN

Although I had experienced what I thought of as significant pain at other times in my life, until I awoke from surgery I had never really understood *terrible pain*, pain that morphine and Demerol can't touch, pain on which none of the usual tricks for evading or even embracing pain provide significant relief, pain during which there is no life, no feeling, no thought—only pain. I did not know that a human being can feel such pain and remain conscious.

Terrible pain is not easy to describe to those who have not experienced it—no easier, I suppose, than explaining colors to the blind, melody to the deaf, deep depression to those who are not temperamentally prone to it (William Styron's noble failure to do so in *Darkness Visible* bears this out), or the fourth or fifth dimension to those of us accustomed to dealing with only three. To attempt this description is, I am afraid, to attempt explanation of the unexplainable. Nevertheless I will try.

Imagine an explosion inside your body that goes off not once, but continually, at unpredictable intervals; and imagine that each time you start to adjust to the shock of one explosion, astonished that somehow you managed to survive it and convinced that you could not do so again, another one hits, even more powerful than the one before. Now imagine this scenario going on for days, no end in sight, the explosions and aftershocks interrupted only by periods of drug-induced blankness that may or may not contain additional explosions of pain.

Another try—

Imagine yourself to be a child in, say, the Nebraska plains during the dust bowl era. There is a tornado brewing, and somehow you have become separated from your clan, who by now are all safely lodged in the storm cellar. You are clinging to the porch rail, partly sheltered by the house itself, and still you feel the wind surge and crash around you, threatening to carry you away. For a moment you consider trying to make it to the shelter, there to wait out the storm with your loved ones, but the force is too ferocious. You venture just one foot off the porch, and then suddenly it is all you can do to hold on. As you struggle to recement your grip, the wind surges again and you feel your body lifted from the wooden planks, your face and frame pelted by bits of grit and debris, and you know that if the next surge is any stronger your grip will fail. Then, inevitably, the next surge *is* stronger, and the house itself is swept away and you are literally flapping in the wind, clinging to the orphaned rail like a flag on a flagpole, the storm doors beneath which your family lies huddled fading to invisibility beneath their mask of dust and debris. And then the wind surges again, even stronger.

Again—

Imagine yourself as a snail clinging to a rock along the shoreline. The tide comes in and the waves crash against you, each one testing the limits of your ability to hold on, each one, you are certain, the maximum force you can withstand, each one stronger than the one before. You let go, contracting as deeply into your shell as you can and still the force of the water crashes against you, crushing you against the rocks, shaking you to your center, forcing you farther in, so that in a short while you are aware of nothing but surviving the beating, bracing yourself for the next blow, knowing that if it is any more vigorous than the last you will have to succumb, finding it, in fact, impossible to imagine a stronger blow; and then discovering with the next, stronger blow that *there is no succumbing*, there is only merciless, unremitting beating and the equally merciless, equally unremitting surviving.

What I have been trying to convey is that after a very short period of being subjected to terrible pain, you can do nothing but endure. There is no room left in the organism for anything resembling conventional consciousness, for a scrap of an idea, for even the most fleeting emotion. There is only the reality of pain, and in my case (but not, I think, in many cases of pain even worse than mine—abdominal pain, though high on the list, is not considered the pinnacle of pain), of periods of dreamy, drug-induced oblivion, the hallucinations finally more real than anything else. My recollections of this period are almost wholly of this brute endurance, endurance against even my own will to lose consciousness to escape it. I was not a human being. I was not even Prufrock's pair of ragged claws, scuttling. I was Pain.

My brother Alan, who called me from Switzerland during this period, told me later that he thought I had lost my mind. A friend of mine, after hearing my tale, told me that my description of the pain following surgery sounded like the pain of giving birth.

Before this incident, I had always thought that pain was not the problem with illness or dying, that with enough pain-control medication any amount of pain could be effectively muted. This is also a common belief among members of the medical profession who speak against doctor-assisted suicide. They say that these patients would not want to die if the quality of their lives could be maintained beyond the savage struggle to endure that I have tried to describe. But issues of dignity notwithstanding (some might choose to end their lives while they were still at least a semblance of their former selves), my experience is that such faith in the efficacy of pain medication is not always warranted.

Of course, I endured this pain for only a few days. It may be that after a longer endurance I would somehow have adapted to these conditions, that my humanity would have emerged (there are such people), but in my case I think not. In my case, particularly if I knew (and you do know) that there would be no remission of this pain, I believe my only thought could be for an end to suffering.

In my more angry moments, I wish I could inflict on the men and women who make judgments on the proper care and management of the sick and dying (most of them in good health and with no trace of significant illness in their histories) an hour of this type of pain. Though there is much to be said in favor of maintaining life above all, one thing that has become clear to me from my own brief exposure is that there are things in life worse than death, and that in some cases death really is the better alternative. I have come to believe that we should have the right to choose that alternative, or to nominate others to make that choice if we ourselves are helpless to carry it out.

THE HOSPITAL

The 12 days following surgery was a hazy, disorienting time.

The hospital was my world. I had no sense of the scale of my environment. At first, I was aware only of my half of the room, and that only dimly. When I walked for the first time past my roommate's bed and finally into the hall, a distance of about 10 feet, I felt as if I were walking down an endless corridor. And only when I came back from that walk and saw the room from a vertical position did I have any sense of the geometry of the space I'd been inhabiting for the previous 3 or 4 days.

Though I could still talk during this period, I couldn't really remember, and the talking and responding felt automatic, disconnected from who and where I was. Inside, I was still mostly this creature from the Waiting Room, holed up in a shell that protected me from the hurricane going on outside, in my body.

I did not wash or shave for 10 days, could not eat or drink for more than a week, did not brush my teeth, and did not notice that I did not do these things. I didn't care about the world outside. The television images on the news were the same as the television images in *Star Trek*.

But I was not apathetic. Early in my recovery, I remember staring out the window at the hospital wall in the gray Syracuse afternoon, tubes flowing in, tubes flowing out, immobile, and I remember understanding at last how a quadriplegic could still feel he had something to live for. Though nearly as helpless, I was still alive, and I wanted to know what would happen next.

As time passed I gradually began to unfold, to break through from inside to outside, like a bean sprouting. With the removal of each tube I felt more human. I became cognizant of the whole room and the man with whom I shared it. I became more mobile, able to navigate on my own. Soon, my world encompassed not only the room but also the hallway, and a few days later, the whole floor. After a while, like a child impatient with the confines of his playpen, I wanted to go to other floors, to see the cafeteria, though the nurses, like overprotective parents, wouldn't let me.

When I was off the heaviest pain killers and all but one of the tubes were gone, I finally felt a little like me. In the 10 days since my near-death experience, many of the little pieces of me that had been stripped away by the rush to death had begun to coalesce around the core that had always been there, but of whose existence, until I was dying, I had never been aware.

After the worst of the pain had subsided, I also felt that I had gained from this experience more than I had lost; that in a few days I had insights into the nature of death and life that I could have learned only after decades of meditation and study, if then.

Though I would not have chosen this path to knowledge, I nevertheless felt lucky I had stumbled on it. Now, after much continuing illness and the prospect of living my life with the unresolved consequences of this event, I am less sure, but a friend of mine who went through a somewhat similar disaster a few years before me says that the feeling of having improved returns once you are finally more or less well. She says that a kind of power slowly develops, which she believes stays with you the rest of your life.

I hope she is right.

BEDPANS

Like infancy, hospital life revolves around eating, drinking, excreting.

The period during which my bowels first began to function remains one of the more vivid memories of my postsurgical period. This is partly because it was then that I experienced the second greatest pain, pain at times equal to the postoperative pain, though of much briefer duration. But it is vivid mostly because of the ascent it marked from the embryonic state of surgery into a second infancy.

The most notable indicator of this second infancy was the bedpan.

I remember clearly—and I have told no one this—the moment when I passed my first bowel movement since the surgery, a bowel movement of blood. My patched-together intestines had begun to wake themselves from their long, injured sleep the day before, with loud bowel sounds and, some hours later, a small amount of passed gas. I was alone and in too much pain to get to the bathroom by myself or locate my bedpan (which, I also realized at that moment, I did not know precisely how to use), and though I pressed the nurse's call button, I felt my own call too urgently to wait the usual 15 or 20 minutes between the time I rang and the time someone came to help. So I let whatever was to happen happen, hoping feebly that this was merely more gas.

Afterward, as I waited for assistance, I remembered visiting my Uncle Morrie, my father's oldest brother, a few months before he died in a ward in the Veterans Administration hospital in Cleveland. On that visit, he, too, had shat himself, and my brother Alan and I had tried to help clean him up, finally abandoning him to a nurse when the task overwhelmed us. "I hope I'm dead before that happens to me," I had said, and Alan said he felt the same way. But when I found myself in a similar state of helplessness, being dead was not at all what I wanted. I wanted more life.

"I thought it was just a fart," I told Yvonne, the sour-faced patient assistant who, a few days later when she broke my shaving mirror, would panic at the thought of 7 years' bad luck. As Yvonne cleaned me up, I found that, unlike the unredeemable shame I have felt in dreams in which this has happened, I felt instead a kind of relief, an unburdening as emotional as it was physical. I had done the most socially disgraceful thing I could imagine, and it had meant nothing much to anyone.

When Yvonne replaced my pad, I noticed that the soiled one was burgundy red, and a wave of panic swept through me. By then I had been on some combination of morphine, Valium, and Demerol for almost a week, and the drugs had started to affect my mind. I hallucinated frequently, and I was, if not actually paranoid, then at least highly suspicious. I called the nurse, who reassured me that this was merely "old blood," exactly as the other nurse had said the week before. I became convinced that I was bleeding again. I thought, "This is like in horror movies, when just as the hero declares that the monster is dead and buried, a hand reaches out from the grave and pulls you under."

As soon as the nurse left the room I called my brother Steven, who, because of his many business contacts in the Cleveland community, was the one person I believed I could count on to handle what I perceived to be a new emergency.

"Steve?" I said. At this point I still had a tube running down my throat and my voice was a vague croak.

"Dave?"

"Yeah. Steve, I think I'm bleeding again."

"Oh, shit. What's going on?"

"I just moved my bowels for the first time and it was all blood."

"Have you seen the doctor? What does he say?"

"He's not around. The nurse said it was old blood, but that's what they said to me a week ago, and they were wrong. She said she'd get the surgeon in here, but I don't know if I can trust him. He's an asshole."

"Yeah, Rick said he was a real charmer."

"Really? I didn't even know they met. Anyway, Steve, I don't know what to do. I don't trust these people. If they screwed up the first time, I don't want them mucking around inside me again. They almost killed me before. This time they might."

"Right." He was silent, but I could hear muffled voices in the background. "It's David," he said to the voices. "He thinks he's bleeding again."

"Jesus," he said to me.

"Steve, if I need more surgery, I want to go somewhere else. Can you find a way to get me to a hospital in Cleveland?"

More silence. "Shit, Dave, I don't know what to do."

More muffled voices. "We'll figure out something. Maybe we can helicopter you in or something. I'll talk to Mom and Dad. Don't worry. Hang in there. If you're afraid these people are butchers and they're going to hurt you, somehow, trust me, we'll get you here."

Later, Steven confided, "I was concerned. I wasn't freaked out. But what I didn't like was this feeling—and I don't like it in any situation—this feeling of helplessness. I didn't know what the hell to do. Because my theory was, if we make the wrong decision, maybe we're gonna kill him. You know?"

When the surgeon came by about an hour later, he explained (as, unbeknownst to me, he had already told my brother Rick) that there had been "a gallon of blood" in my intestines, and he had left it there. This blood-expelling process would continue for some days, and this time, I understood, it really was "expected."

Over the next couple of days, I was wracked by frequent bouts of diarrhea, the several days' accumulation of methane produced by rotting blood gradually expanding my stapled-together intestines and then emptying them.

During these episodes, I would experience pain nearly as extreme as that which immediately followed surgery, though it was of shorter duration. First there was the pain of trapped liquids and gasses pressing against recently torn-up tissue, then a wave during which all I could do was howl and frantically adjust the position of the bed as my bowels emptied into the pan. The pain lasted for perhaps 2 or 3 minutes, then the spasm passed. Half an hour later, the same thing would happen again, and this cycle would repeat perhaps six times in a row, until finally everything that was in me was out.

Sometimes Yvonne would clean me up and then empty the bedpan, handling me almost as if I were a newborn and she a reluctant nanny; at other times it was Stephanie, an attractive redhead who taught aerobics when she wasn't nursing; and when neither nurse nor patient assistant was handy, it was Hatsune or, the Saturday following surgery, my former girlfriend Sylvia, who had come in from Boston to spend the day caring for me. In terms of modesty it no longer mattered to me who did what, though I did rank each of my caretakers in terms of their thoroughness and gentleness. I preferred the touch of more familiar hands, who also did a better job of cleansing.

When I left the hospital, I left to my mother's care, as I had from another hospital nearly 41 years before. Unlike my father, who commemorated my baths, haircuts, and first steps in snapshots and 8-millimeter home movies, I don't have a visual record of these reiterated childhood events. But my damaged memory does recall, like pages in a disordered scrapbook, the first time Sylvia got me walking, being sponge-bathed by 80-year-old Millie Schreiber, the time Stephanie washed my hair, the first time I managed to use a toilet, my first solid food.

I remember the interminable drive back from the hospital to my apartment, and I remember especially the first time I was able to walk to the end of my block. I lived in the country at the time, and the block was half a mile long. When I reached the highway, I stood uncertainly for several minutes, like a child whose mother has told him he could not cross the street, before I finally stepped out onto the road and over to the other side.

My Mother, My Father, My Illness

Those who cannot remember the past are condemned to repeat it.

George Santayana

The cycle of reliving your life that begins with the near-death experience does not end when you leave the hospital. Near-death gives you a chance to live your life over again, sometimes making the same mistakes, sometimes making new ones, but also, sometimes, correcting what went wrong the first time around.

I think what happens is something like the process I've been observing in my friend Janice and her daughter. Like me, Janice was an emotionally abused child. Now she has a child of her own, and in the 8 years of Kimberly's life I have often seen Janice on the verge of repeating her past, about to become her mother in exactly the way that caused her own childhood to be traumatic. But most of the time, out of some combination of love and psychotherapy, Janice manages to short-circuit the bad stuff and to invent within herself the mother she would like to have had, the mother who does the right thing. As she soothes or cajoles Kimberly, at the same time, it is as if the shattered child in her is shadowing her own child; the process of doing right by her daughter seems to heal Janice's old wounds. As she mothers Kim, I have seen Janice transform into the healthier version of her adult self that she might more easily have been if she had had a mother as capable as she.

Coming back from near-death, I have found myself soothing and cajoling and fathering the wounded parts of me. Though I haven't had the tangible example of an actual child to attend to, I have had help.

———■———

In a dream I had about 6 years ago, I criticized my mother's cooking, said something harsh about a spinach dish she had prepared; I don't remember the details. My tone was argumentative, and I think it was that tone, rather than the specific criticism, she responded to. In the dream, her reaction was extreme: instantaneously enraged, she stabbed me through the heart with a hat pin. As I staggered back, I saw that the wound left no blood, though I knew, just before I awoke, that it would be fatal.

Like Sisters' Hospital, my mother was both life-bearing and life-threatening.

One of the few gifts of my recent tangle with death and sickness has been that most of the scars from my childhood have finally been, like the umbilical remnant the surgeons removed, expunged. Years of grappling, as well as interviews with uncles and aunts who observed our family dynamic when I was young, had helped me to recon-struct the ways in which both of my parents, especially my mother, were themselves made unhappy by their marriage, and this has made it easier to accept the things that were done to me, or not done for me, by them. But though I acknowledged these things in my mind a decade ago, and though my day-to-day life has for years been relatively unaffected by childhood trauma, until I approached death's gates, the deepest pain remained as fresh as it was when the wounds were first inflicted.

Like the children of alcoholic mothers or fathers—the "adult children," as they call themselves—I still exhibit a well-defined set of neuroses. But I'm not hurt by what my mother did to me anymore. I've forgiven her for my childhood. That pain has been wiped clean.

I'm not sure why.

One possible explanation is that the actual site in my brain where the hurt was stored has been wiped clean, too. According to the neurologist and the neuropsycholo-gist I consulted, I suffered diffuse brain damage, primarily on the left side, due to lack of oxygen during extended periods of extremely low blood pressure. Since then, much healing has taken place—the brain, like the heart, is a resilient organ—and extensive testing has revealed only one remaining weak area: memory. So perhaps along with mental maps of the streets of Somerville and Cambridge, Massachusetts; some dozens of names, compound words, and faces; and the content of the many books, movies, and conversations I'll never know I no longer remember, the memories of that hurt—the residues of that pain—were destroyed as well.

Or perhaps it was (and this is the theory I favor) just that when my mother came to take care of me, she had a chance to mother me all over again, and this time she suc-ceeded in being kind where she had been cruel, thoughtful where she had been selfish, loving where she had been hateful, loyal where she had betrayed me. Whatever the cause, the burden of my childhood has been lifted, the child in me has been released, and for the first time in my adult life I am free to love my mother again.

I see no sign of this ending while she and I both live.

As soon as my family heard what had happened to me, my mother and my brother Richard made plans to visit: my mother was to come first, and then a few days later my brother. When they presented this plan to me just before I was shipped down to the ICU, I asked that the order be reversed. I wanted Richard there as close as he could be to the surgery; as a medical person himself, I felt I could count on Richard to under-stand my best interests and to represent them to the doctors. My mother was to come to Syracuse after I was released from the hospital, when I suspected (accurately, it turned out) I would need a great deal of care.

This is the story I asked Hatsune to tell my mother during the time I came out of my near-death experience and the time I left for the ICU. But it wasn't, I think, the *whole* story. I believe that in the back of my mind there was also the recollection that when-ever there has been trouble in my life or in the lives of any of my brothers, my mother's reaction more often added to the problem than helped to relieve it. I must have known even then that if I survived the night I would have enough problems of my own to deal with, without having to cope with her panic or insecurities as well.

Ten days later, when I called from the hospital to confirm my mother's trip to Syracuse, I was far from optimistic about our enduring each other's presence in what I knew would be intimate quarters and stressful conditions. I lived some 20 miles outside of the city, in a one-bedroom apartment. I also drove a stick-shift car; although she had driven one throughout my childhood and adolescence, my mother claimed she could no longer operate a stick-shift. For a week or two, we would be thrown together more tightly than we'd been since I was an infant, and I would be nearly as dependent on her as I was then, and even more isolated. Although periods of sickness were the only times, as a child, I had gotten her full attention, in my adult life my most recent experience of being seriously ill—a ruptured disk in the lumbar region of my spine, for which I'd spent a month in bed in a rigid brace at my parents' house 12 years before—taught me that my mother had little tolerance for me as a sick adult. At that time, my despair only made her impatient, and her impatience quickly turned to anger directed against me. I predicted—and so did both she and my brothers—that I would send her home or she would flee before the first week was over.

But as it turned out she stayed 2 weeks, the second against my father's wishes, and by being, at 70, a good mother to me, she managed to undo, apparently permanently, the residual harm that still haunted me from childhood.

When I was a child, my mother's needs always came before ours, and the consequences of ignoring them were severe. Although she was often careless about birthday presents for us—she got us what *she* liked or what was on sale—if we forgot an anniversary or a birthday, she flew into a crying fit or a rage. This time, when I was as a child again, she took care of things with what was for me, from her, unprecedented efficiency and compassion. She thought of my needs first and seemed mostly to disregard her own, which was exactly what I needed at the time.

She was really quite wonderful. She mobilized my kitchen, entertained my friends when they came to visit, and the night before my 42nd birthday, in what they now call the blizzard of '92, when my fever suddenly jumped 3 degrees in 2 hours and the water turned brackish because the pipe from the pump had sprung a leak, she introduced herself to my neighbors, assured me she would find a way to get me to the hospital if I needed to, obtained a few days' supply of bottled water, and in general . . . handled things.

She also kept me entertained. She had brought with her a bunch of old movies and 10 hours of *The Outer Limits* (I am still a science fiction fan and, next to *Twilight Zone* and *Star Trek*, this was my favorite show). These films and episodes kept me going when she and I were stranded in my apartment, before she finally ventured out in my car into the snow-choked streets for food and more movies.

When it became clear that she would be taking care of me for more than a couple of days she recruited one of my visitors to teach her how to drive my car. After one chaperoned test drive to the local supermarket, she became my chauffeur, the two of us managing to make the 20-mile trip into town over bumpy potholes that shook my shattered body, she driving and me coaching her on braking, shifting, and directions, as if we were symbionts who together formed one person who could drive a stick-shift car. Once she was mobile, she sought out the store that gave triple coupons and the one with the best produce, stocked my refrigerator and freezer with precooked meals for a month, and labeled and indexed the frozen packages. By the time she left she had collected $20 or $30 worth of coupons and convinced me I should use them. (I still don't, but Hatsune does, "for the sake of your mother.")

However, my mother's most impressive feat occurred as the first week drew to a close. Although it was evident to both of us that I would not be able to manage on my own if she left at the end of that week, she and I both also knew that my father wanted her back. His calls, rather than expressing concern about my state of health, urged me to return to Cleveland, where, as he put it, they could "all take care of me," and more importantly where my mother could take care of him. Though his health has been compromised by two heart attacks and various lesser ailments and he would, in fact, die the following year, at that time he seemed in no danger and was not in any obvious way impaired. (He swam every day at the Jewish Center, and later that year he and my mother would take a Caribbean cruise.) Yet he had become accustomed to my mother's care, and with each call he sounded more helpless. Toward the end of the first week I also began to get calls from my brothers in Cleveland attesting to his weakening mental condition.

"Dad's really falling apart without Mom," my brother Steve told me. "The first couple of days, he'd call maybe once or twice. Yesterday he called me five times. He's okay physically, but he's an emotional wreck. I don't know how much longer he can take it. Or how much more *I* can take." My brother's solution, like my father's, was that I return to Cleveland, where my mother could soothe my father and still take care of me. But at that time I was already suffering from worrisome and incapacitating postoperative complications and was still bedridden except for brief walks and meals. I was in no shape to travel the 6 hours by train or even the 2 hours by taxi and airplane; and like my father, I did not want to be far from the doctors and nurses who knew my condition.

My mother got on the phone with my brother. After she hung up, I asked what she was going to do. She looked away. "I don't know, David," she said, and then walked into the kitchen to start supper.

In my late teenage years, when I began to come out of my shell by growing my hair long, starting an underground magazine, experimenting with drugs, sex, and politics, my father acted swiftly and sternly to repress me. My mother took the role of my confidant and defendant in these conflicts, or so it seemed, and thus armed, I would sometimes stand up to him. But inevitably, once the conflict became explicit and my father laid down the law, she would switch sides and support him against me. Even in recent years, when my father and I disagreed, her usual pattern would be to interrupt the fight, ostensibly to protect my father. "You're going to give him another heart attack!" she would scream in the middle of our arguments, terminating them abruptly.

I fully expected my mother to follow the same pattern this time and to go back to Cleveland and leave me on my own, or at best under Hatsune's part-time care. But for the first time in my adult life she sized up the situation and decided *I* was the one who needed her most; my father would have to wait. She helped me through the worst of the crisis, and in the end went home to a husband who, despite his complaints and pleas, was none the worse. She gave me, finally, the uncompromised and unconditional love I'd never had as a child, even at the expense of my father's demands. This, as much as anything else, had a healing power.

Shortly before my father's death, my mother and I talked both about the way she handled my illness and about the choices she has made in her own life. About me, she said she did what any parent would have done. I said maybe so, but I was glad she could be a good parent for me. "Finally," she said.

About herself, she told me she would have waited to get married had she the chance to do things differently, and she would have finished college. But she has made her own peace with her choices. "I was in love with him and I wanted to get married, and that's what I did," she said. "You can't look back, David." She is a stronger, wiser woman than the woman who raised me, and part of that strength and wisdom seems to have come from accepting, caring for, and even loving my father again, who, after the rest of us had long since left the nest, was her one remaining child.

Aftershocks

Having come reasonably close to stepping into the shoes I wore before my near-death experience, I find they no longer quite fit who I am now. It's hard to summarize the changes.

Some of them were transitory. For the first several months, I felt possessed of a powerful energy I had never experienced before. I knew who was calling when the phone rang, and letters with infrequent correspondents crossed in the mail. I felt as if I literally had a power I could direct with my hands, like bolts of electricity issuing forth from my palms and fingers. My friend Jay, who is a bit of a psychic himself, told me that if he could see my aura, he was sure it would have been of a different color. As I became increasingly involved in the activities of daily life, however, this psychic sense gradually faded.

Other changes seem to have become a permanent part of my character.

One, common to almost all those who experience near-death, is that I no longer fear death itself. In near-death (and, by extrapolation, in death itself), I think you find the answer to the question you've most been looking for. Although mine wasn't one of the blissful near-death experiences I have since read about, neither was it at all frightening; it was, rather, by far the calmest moment of my life, deeply centering.

Another, which seems to date from the moment of dying itself, is that I am less attached to my physical form and to my past. It is as if the real "I" is a puppeteer manipulating this body, these patterns of behavior.

Having survived a moment when everything I once had planned came abruptly to a halt, I find I now care less about long-term planning than I had before, am more interested in discovering what's out beyond the boundaries of my current life, am willing to take more risks.

Other changes are more general. My friends tell me I am somewhat more patient in little things, more tolerant than I was before of other people's foibles and of my own. On the other hand, I tend not to cooperate in other people's plans unless they fit into mine and am much more immune to guilt and shame. I spend more time writing and thinking and less time worrying about what it will amount to. I find it almost impossible to lie.

My mind seems also to have changed. I find abstract thinking both less interesting and more difficult, while imaginative thinking and writing is easier. Testing has borne out this subjective impression: Although my total IQ score 3 months after my near-death experience was the same as it had been the year before, a previously substantial divergence between my ability to perform right- and left-brain tasks had evened out, as if the rough edges of my mind had been sanded smooth.

These changes I regard, for the most part, as positive.

The benefits of changes due to the radical surgery and my continuing illnesses, on the other hand, for the most part elude me.

Though the subtext of much of the story I have been telling, despite the sometimes horrific nature of the details, is generally positive, this is not the reaction I get when I talk about it to friends or family who have not seen me since all this occurred. When they ask me, "What's new?" and I tell them my story, the reaction I get is almost always, "You've been through hell, haven't you?"

If I look at how things have gone compared to how they might have had I never come close to death, I see that in many ways this experience has shattered me, has left me with damages in all of the major areas of my life. Although the near-death experience itself was uplifting, that lift came at a cost, and the cost has been dear. The impact of the initial hemorrhaging and the aftereffects of bungled surgery have ruined me financially, nearly destroyed my relationship with Hatsune, and left me with numerous physical, mental, and emotional injuries, some of which may never fully heal.

Despite what I have gained in wisdom and insight, had I to do it over again, I would not. I often wonder what would have happened to me if I had never gone to the hospital at all. I had been bleeding for two days, and in two more days I stopped. Perhaps, as the ER doctor warned me, in a few more days I would have bled massively and died before I made it to the operating room. Or perhaps the injury would have healed on its own, never to trouble me again. I'll never know. Either way, my fate would have been a good deal more clear than my life has been since that crisp Saturday afternoon when I took myself to the Sisters' Hospital emergency room.

GRIEF

Although I may ultimately require more surgery with its own burden of pain, I sense that the greatest pain I have yet to fully experience is emotional, not physical.

For the first several weeks after my near-death experience, every morning I woke up thinking about the moments before dying and the people I would have lost had I died. Each time it was someone else—my brother Rick, my mother, my friend Olga, Hatsune—and each time I would begin to cry, uncontrollably, as if it were they who would have died, not me. Sylvia, my former girlfriend, told me she cried on the way home from visiting me at Sisters' Hospital, realizing that I could have died but then telling herself no, I couldn't die, I was part of her world. What I felt is something like that, but I felt it for each of them: that I couldn't die and lose them, they are part of my world.

This aspect of the grieving process has strengthened me, stabilized me. But it was frequently interrupted—in the hospital by the ministrations of the nurses, doctors, and hospital staff and at home by phone calls, visits, interactions with my caretakers. By the time I began to reenter daily life, there was still much grieving left to do. Though I'm not really sure exactly what I have left to grieve for, I know that in addition to the people I almost lost, I have yet to fully grieve for my lost intestines, my dead brain cells, my ravaged life. Or even for the old life I left behind that I don't seem to be able to live anymore.

Like anything else that is held in, grief repressed finds another, subtler exit.

According to a brochure I picked up in the office of the neuropsychologist who tested me for brain damage, post-traumatic stress disorder (PTSD) results from exposure to an event "outside the range of usual human experience." The brochure lists the indicators that identify one who suffers from this disorder:

> 1) intrusive symptoms such as replaying or reexperiencing the traumatic event in dreams or in an awake state; 2) distancing symptoms such as a decrease in responsiveness, a constriction of affect, loss of interest in activities, withdrawal from others, and avoidance of situations and people associated with the trauma; and 3) symptoms related to heightened autonomic reactions, such as startle responses, irritability, and hypervigilance. Disruptions in close interpersonal relationships are common.

A later paragraph mentions that it is common for adult sufferers to relive childhood traumas. A sidebar lists possible inciting incidents: "Car accidents, plane crash, combat, armed robbery, battering, witnessing trauma, fires, rape, childhood sexual assault, construction accidents, cult participation, on-the-job injury." Oddly missing was my particular trauma, near-fatal bleeding and major emergency surgery.

In Virginia Woolf's *Mrs. Dalloway*, shell-shocked Septimus Warren Smith thinks and talks of how he cannot feel. His inability to feel, *we* feel, is ultimately what drives him to suicide. Though a more general term, "post-traumatic stress disorder" seems far less descriptive than the much older term for the problem that was current in Woolf's time. "Shell-shocked" seems to describe both the origin and result: having been among the shells when they exploded, having one's feelings packed into a shell, and finally becoming a shell of one's former self.

In my case the onset of PTSD occurred when I reached the point where I could more or less care for myself but had not yet sufficiently grieved. By now, my "heightened autonomic reactions"—being startled almost out of my chair each time the phone rang or panicked each time another car came too close—have calmed, but I'm still much more sensitive than I was before. By now, writing and group therapy have helped me to neutralize the waking part of the "intrusive symptoms," the waking reliving. But the experience still thrives in my dreams.

The dreams come less often now. In the first year, however, there were at least a hundred nights from which I woke soaked in sweat, heart racing. Only a dozen or so of the dreams themselves survived into waking consciousness, and of these I now recall only a few, primarily those I wrote down. By any previous standards I might have called all of these dreams nightmares, but I find it hard to classify them as such because my actual experience was nearly as traumatic, sometimes more so.

A sampling:

1. A demonstration

I am to be part of a surgical demonstration that my brother Richard is directing. I am on an operating table, along with another subject whose table is at the opposite side of the surgical theater. I notice that a rather large audience has gathered around us, perhaps 12 or 15 young men and women, presumably medical students.

First, my brother shows the two interns who will perform the surgeries how the procedure should be done. He demonstrates on another patient, or perhaps it is a cadaver. He makes two vertical slits, one on each side of the mid-torso, each halfway between the hips and belly button. The slits are perhaps 2 inches long, and they go just through the skin, no deeper. A clear fluid seeps from the wounds and then quickly stops, a fluid that resembles drainage from a wound.

The interns then begin their activities. Working in parallel, these student surgeons simultaneously cut into both me and the other patient. I know immediately that my cuts go much too deep: I can see my bleeding flesh like a slab of cut meat and beneath it my blood-swathed organs. My heart races, but I trust that my brother will be able to remedy this error.

Richard is still talking about the procedure. I call him over, and my intern calls him, too, in a panic about the blood. Then I become aware that the intern on the opposite side of the room has made the same mistake, and that Richard, who I know could save me, is also called to help him. As I feel my life seep out, I realize that although Richard is good at what he does, he is not good enough to save us both. Richard, helpless to choose between us, continues to lecture, moving back and forth between me and the other dying patient, appraising and describing the terrible situation he can do nothing to reverse.

2. A do-it-yourself job

I'm in some kind of a war, in Britain. I'm from Madrid, but I'm in a military hospital and surgery is being performed on me. In the midst of the operation, the hospital is hit with a shell. The medical staff scatters, leaving me alone in the operating theater. I am conscious through all this but am afraid to move lest my exposed organs spill out. Eventually, in an act of desperation, knowing that I have little chance of getting it right but knowing as well that the alternative is probably to bleed to death before anyone returns to help me, I sew up the organs, close the muscle walls myself.

Somehow I complete the job, but I leave a needle inside me. Some time later, the doctors tell me I shouldn't have closed the incision myself, but I explain that I had to, I couldn't stay perfectly still while I waited for them to return. "I'm amazed that the whole thing worked," I tell them, and they nod reluctant agreement. I tell them I'm going back to Madrid, and they ask me if I need anything for home. The nurse looks on sympathetically. I say, "No, I have everything I need." And then I start choking on my own blood, which is pouring out through my nose.

When I wake up, I feel overwhelmingly sad. I feel as if I'll never be safe, and until I realize I've been dreaming, I'm convinced that this time the bleeding won't stop. This time, I will die.

3. Shoot-out

This dream followed a discussion in which I talked about all the hardware that they left in me, the stitches and the staples.

I'm in the middle of a gun battle in a large department store. Crouched with me behind couches and tables tumbled into a makeshift barrier is a sort of cowboy, like the character Jack Palance plays in *City Slickers*, and several soldiers. I don't see who they're shooting at, but during the gunplay I'm shot in the ankle and the bullet lodges there. I see it, a silver cylinder surrounded by red, swollen flesh, flush with the surface of my skin. We debate about whether to take it out or leave it in. The cowboy and the soldiers decide it's probably better to leave it in because I'd bleed too much if they took it out.

I try to walk on my injured leg, and my ankle shatters.

4. Amputation

A more recent dream. In it, I wake up in a hospital room. I'm all right, they tell me, except that they had to amputate both my arms just above the elbow. They've fitted me with prosthetic limbs that seem to be alive. Sometime later I am sitting in a bar with my brother Steve and we talk this over. "This doesn't make any sense," I say. "What could've been wrong that they had to cut off *both* my arms?"

Later in the dream, I discuss the situation with my mother. "Don't you know?" she says, sobbing. "She gave you bad blood. She didn't check it first."

I wake up with a start and shake my arms to be certain they are real.

5. Sanitarium

I am in a sanitarium. I have some kind of fatal disease that it appears everybody else there also has, though mine may kill me quicker. It's a rare disease; I can't remember now how it kills.

For a while I am apparently in some kind of denial, but at some point during my stay in the sanitarium I understand that death might actually overtake me. I talk with a young woman I've just met who also has the disease. I tell her, crying a little, that I haven't had anyone to talk to about it, that I've been holding it all inside. She turns away, but I tell her that I won't unburden everything on her, I just need to talk, and she says okay.

"Maybe I won't grow old," I tell her. "Maybe I'll never have a kid." That's the thing, I tell her, I'll most regret, never having had a kid.

And so on.

More troubling for me than the dreams has been the "distancing" mentioned in the PTSD brochure. Beneath what by now must appear a fairly ordinary surface I sometimes still find myself in a state of curious numbness, a condition in which I cannot fully love, hate, or fear, at least not during my waking hours. Though not without its own delights, it is a shadowy, frustrating sort of existence in which the familiar passions, along with the unresolved terrors of the original inciting incident, are buried together, presumably until the sufferer in me is somehow coaxed out of hiding, can be convinced that life is actually a reasonably safe place in which to grieve.

Life often feels much as it did when I was a child, when nobody would take care of me, soothe me. Now, as then, I've figured out how to take care of myself, but I still sometimes feel shattered inside and wish I could just cry until I was better. But you have to feel very safe in order to cry about things like this.

DEFORMITY

In addition to the emotional damage, there is also a physical legacy.

In a number of ways surgery has left me different from the way I was and different from most of the people I know. The differences are mostly invisible unless you know me well, under the clothing and under the skin, but some of them are fairly obvious. I have a 12-inch incision, a pale red band now about a quarter of an inch wide that drops from my breastbone straight down my midline, detours to the right around my belly button, and then continues on its original path until it reaches my groin.

The scar itself has a number of unusual features, all of them now a part of me. Beneath its surface in the first inch or so I (or you; anybody, really) can still feel the stitches underneath, permanently embedded in the slab of scar tissue where fascia and muscle used to be. Part of this subcutaneous tissue, the part sutured to my breastbone with a great nylon knot (since removed), has calcified into something currently about halfway between cartilage and bone. From time to time the ersatz joint between this neo-bone and my breastbone makes a disconcerting pop, almost precisely like a knuckle coming in and out of joint.

Farther down, the external scar deepens in color, and beneath it is a wide, softer slab perhaps 3 inches in diameter. This is where they patched the original incision with nylon mesh when, a few months after the initial operation, a large hole appeared in my abdominal wall where the wound had been infected. Just below that patch is a glob of fat cells that was originally 3 or 4 inches lower, and below that is the hollow where the fat cells used to be. When they stitched me back together, they displaced this tissue; though the surgeon promised me it would eventually join its twin on my other side, this promise of a return to normality has turned out to be as empty as several of his others.

Here and there are various subtle defects, small hernias perhaps the size of the tip of your (or mine; anybody's, really) finger. Fatty tissue protrudes through them. They cause me pain when I cough, sneeze, or lift more than about 25 pounds, and they may in time require yet another surgery, this time to replace the entire incision, thus creating a new foot-long scar and new potential for yet another set of hernias, another patch, another scar—a cycle that I fear could, in the worst case, continue ad infinitum. Two of these defects pop to the touch, something like the clicking crickets and frogs kids used to get as birthday party favors. One of the hernias slowly but steadily increases in size, making further surgery likely.

At the bottom of the incision, invisible and inaccessible to the touch, is a large nylon knot tied to my pubic bone. It shifts as my musculature attempts to adapt to my new internal arrangement and pulls on the nerves of my groin or lower abdomen for a day or two before it settles down again. Deeper still, beneath the ravaged abdominal wall, is a cavity where some 2 or 3 feet of large intestine used to be. A pair of steel staple lines form a new, jerry-rigged connection between my truncated small and large bowels. These connections, composed of many small staples, are evident to me only through the intense pain they caused the first week or so following surgery and the chronic diarrhea that is the legacy of having removed the bowel tissue.

When I try to do a sit-up, the whole scarred mess beneath the skin rises to the surface of my belly as if it were a snake writhing within me, trying to get out. My friend Jay, who is a psychotherapist, asked me to tell him what my scar would look like if it were a person. I told him it would be a burned and crippled wreck of a man. He asked me what it would say if it could talk. I told him it would say, "Let me die."

I know that my deformities are small relative to those who have lost limbs, for example, or whose faces have been hideously rearranged by cancer or the windshield of a car, and I know things could have been worse: I could have died, or been left incontinent. But such deformities are conspicuously absent from most of my friends and family, particularly those my age and younger, and they are, anyway, not small to me. Sometimes, they seem to highlight the other differences I sense between myself and those around me. My scarred belly reifies a sense of deformity and alienation I had as a child and had carried with me most of my life—though, curiously, most of the psychic wounds of my childhood vanished during my recovery from this more tangible injury, as if that life of hidden wounds ended and a new one, where the damage was visible, began. As a child my deformity was my Jewishness, my intelligence, my shyness, my awkwardness, my vulnerability. Now it is the nature of my illness and the closeness with which it brought me to death.

In both cases the feeling is of being irrevocably and irretrievably damaged, now literally branded as somehow not fit for ordinary human company. To the extent that the deformities are invisible, to the extent that the deformed person can "pass," they are all the more shameful, are dark secrets waiting to be revealed, to be the cause of scorn or derision. They are something that *must* be hidden away because they *are* hidden.

I have become an expert on a subject very few of the people I know wish to talk about. For example, at a party shortly after my illness—it was my first social appearance, really; I was still too weak to drive—a woman I had until that moment thought of as potentially a close friend interrupted my telling of what had happened by saying, "You know, it's like a woman trying to describe what it's like to have a baby. No matter how much you talk about it, nobody else can really understand it unless it happened to them." I had been to her house many times and played with her children. We had worked side by side, and she had even tried to play matchmaker between me and another of her friends, but my attempt to recount for her, even if inadequately, what at the time seemed to me the most important single event of my life was too threatening for her to allow me to complete it.

My downstairs neighbor, an outdoorsy kind of guy who used to go out of his way to chat when we ran into each other in the parking lot, after my illness went equally as much out of his way to avoid me until the pallor left my cheeks and the limp went out of my walk. Many of my colleagues managed to stay clear of me throughout my entire recovery, and they will now discuss only the ordinary superficialities of work life. It is as if they fear even the commonplace, "How are you feeling?" because my answer might not be, "Fine."

Illness, and closeness to death, has been a kind of watershed for who I number among my friends and who I relegate, perhaps forever, to acquaintanceship. The people on either side of that equation are not the same as I might have thought before. Now, the ones I find I am most able to talk with are those who believed I might have something of value to tell them, who treated me as if I were a correspondent from another world, as I suppose I am. They have almost all either been with a loved one through a long illness or themselves been close to death. But many others will at least listen, even if they make no claims to fully understand, and most of the time, that is enough.

The fear of those who avoid me is now more frustrating than it is alienating. Because I do have something to tell them about death, something that might comfort them to know.

Reflections

REVISITING SISTERS' HOSPITAL

For 2 weeks—2 weeks that on the one hand stretched into nearly infinite time and on the other are largely eradicated from my active memory—Sisters' Hospital was both my womb and my incubator. Perhaps that is why, despite near-fatal medical errors per-petrated there that have left me with lingering and menacing remnants of disease, I felt some comfort in its presence (but isn't this how we all feel toward mothers who have damaged us?). I have even moved nearby, a 7-minute walk, and though Hatsune and I told ourselves we chose this neighborhood because of its quiet streets, its spaciousness, and our kindly landlords, for me the proximity to Sisters' Hospital was at least uncon-sciously a deciding factor in the move.

A year after my near-death experience I returned to Sisters' Hospital for a visit, as I had once returned to my childhood home long after I had moved away from Cleveland. On this visit, I walked past the room on the fifth floor where I had nearly bled to death; looked briefly into the ICU room in which medical personnel performed tests and infused me with blood and plasma, and toured the sixth floor where I recuperated from surgery.

Paradoxically, as I walked through these now oddly unfamiliar halls, I had the sen-sation of coming home. But as when I returned to the neighborhood of my childhood, the scale was all wrong. Hallway distances that in the early days of my recovery had seemed endless chasms were a few quick steps, had shrunk, much as the block I grew up on had seemed miniaturized when I visited it long after all of my neighbors had died or moved away, after even the square of sidewalk in which several of us kids had left our palm prints had been torn up and repaved.

On entering Sisters' I had felt the anticipation of anxiety being soothed, of happy reunions with some of the hospital staff I had come to think of, while a patient, almost as my friends, as if we had shared intimate relations—had they not inserted tubes into my penis, wiped blood and shit from my ass, entered my body cavity with their knives and instruments, and held my bowels in their hands, palpating them for lumps and lesions? Surely, I thought, being with someone when he is at the boundary of life and death forges a connection, however intangible. But when I saw a couple of the nurses and one of the residents who had worked on me, it took some time for them to recog-nize me, and although they seemed pleased to see that I was doing all right, they also appeared to be embarrassed, talked reluctantly and for only a moment or two. They behaved much as people with whom I'd gone to elementary school or high school have done when I've encountered them on the streets of my home town. Without the context of illness in one case and childhood in the other, we seem to have little to say to one another, and the chance intersection of our otherwise diverged lives is somehow unset-tling for each of us. I remembered earlier visits, when I had returned for tests and vari-ous ministrations, when Sisters' still had that comforting familiarity, a reality more real than my real life, and I thought then that I would miss it when I was well. I took this new strangeness as one more sign that, for better and worse, I am back in the world of the living.

These days, from time to time, I pass hospital personnel on the street and we look at each other quizzically until the moment of mutual recognition finally occurs, and then we move on.

THE JEWEL

When I talked to Sylvia a week or two after I came home from the hospital, I told her I thought my near-death experience was the most important thing that had ever happened to me, and I said I wanted to make a record of it. I told her Hatsune had bought me a small tape recorder for my birthday, and I intended to use it to document what had and would be happening to me. "That's okay," she said, "but the important thing is to get on with your life."

At the time I was irritated by her comment. I felt she was so locked into her narrow, worldly way of doing things that she could not see the significance of this event. Now I'm not so sure.

Coming upon the gifts of a near-death experience is a little like stumbling on a magnificent treasure in a mountain cave. You have traveled far and done perilous things to get there, and you have suffered much, but the trip was worth it. At first you are dazzled and enraptured by the treasure's beauty and power, convinced that its glow will illuminate every portion of your being. You think it will sustain you forever.

In a surprisingly little while, though, you begin to think about your past. At first it is irritating—bothersome calls keep coming in on the cellular phone from friends, family, the business associates who paid for this venture—but in the end, you find you also want to go back home. You wish you could take the treasure with you, but there is no way to get it off the mountain—there is a curse, or it's too heavy, or it's too well guarded. Whatever the reason, try as you might, you just can't do it. So you take just one small jewel.

When you get back home, the whole experience begins to seem dreamlike. Most of your friends are skeptical or uninterested, and soon you begin to doubt any of it ever happened. But you still have the scars from the journey, the lingering pain from where you tumbled down the mountain. And you still have that one small jewel. You look at it from time to time to sustain you, to reassure yourself that the treasure and the rapture were real.

But that jewel doesn't really belong to you, and eventually, perhaps when moving from one apartment to another, you lose that, too. And then all you have left is the residual pain and the scars of the journey and the faded memory of the jewel and the treasure it was part of.

In near-death, I'd felt as if I'd arrived at the end of a spiritual quest. It was a good place to arrive, and I was happy to be there. I thought I'd never feel lonely again. I had found my self.

But I couldn't stay. I couldn't make a religion out of dying. The noisy person I'd been before kept worrying and nagging at me to satisfy its insecurities, to go back to the things I did before and the people with whom I did them. At the time, I resented his noise, and I delayed as long as I comfortably could. Gradually, however, I picked up most of the threads of my earlier life, with each thread and each new compromise feeling that I was losing my hold on the jewel.

For a while I was afraid I would lose something I had nearly died to obtain and might never have a chance to find again. I was constantly torn, trying to choose between the impulses of my old life that were steadily reemerging and the impulses of the life that began that January evening. I thought that if I didn't adhere strictly to the insights and intuitions released during the near-death experience, I would lose everything I'd gained from it, and all I'd have left in the end would be the pain and the loss. The whole struggle, I thought, would have been in vain.

Now I think that the jewel is not so easily discarded.

THE WATCHER

When I was a kid, I read a Marvel comic book called *The Watcher*. The Watcher was a creature as wise and old as the universe. He was always there, looking at what was going on in various corners of inhabited space, reporting with some compassion, but never really interfering. I identified with the Watcher, in the sense that I often felt as if there was a Watcher in me, observing what went on in my chaotic child's life but somehow separate from and unaffected by all it saw.

Years later, when I was in psychotherapy, I understood that this sort of dissociation was how I survived my childhood. I began to perceive that beneath the personality I had acquired as an adult was a small capsule, which I imagined to be cylindrical in shape, its ends tapering gradually to a point. In it, I conjectured, lay my anger, encased in some tough alloy of steel, inaccessible to the me that had grown up around it. As the years passed and I continued treatment, the capsule grew increasingly translucent, and by the time I terminated therapy, I saw the outlines of what I suspected was not my fury, but the shattered remains of a wounded boy.

These days, it has occurred to me that within this capsule, and perhaps within this child as well, was the creature from what I have come to call the Waiting Room, and that that creature is what I now call my self.

Until I attended a support group for people with chronic illness, I did not give much additional thought to this figure, though from time to time he haunted me. Partly in response to a woman who just learned she had cancer and was tormented by fears of dying, I offered to tell of my own encounter with death. After I described the bleeding, the dying, and the coming back, and how I felt about all that, the group's leader dragged a chair in front of me and told me that the creature from my near-death experience was sitting there. "Talk to it," he said.

I went along with the game. "At first," I said to the empty chair in which I could almost imagine that glowing outline of a man-boy, "I felt sure of how to live my life, but now I feel so confused. I thought I'd finally found my way, and now I'm as lost as I ever was. I don't know what to do, and I don't know how to talk to you, or even if you're still there."

The group leader told me to switch chairs. "All right," he said, "now you are the creature and David is sitting there. Answer him."

In my voice, the creature said, "I'm still here, and I'm real and important. But the you that has grown up around me is also real. Both of us live inside you, and you can't choose one or the other. You have to let both of us grow."

Until that moment, I had been attempting to somehow compromise two strong forces inside me, or if I could not compromise, then to choose one over the other. One was this new energy, which I had thought of as my essential self, brought finally into the light from the enclosure it had been sealed into since I was 5 or 10 years old. The other was the self that I had constructed around that enclosure, like rock candy developing around a knotted string.

The literature on near-death experiences claims that compromise is impossible, and that choosing to go on with the new life or return to the old are the only options that can yield happiness and a full life. But now I see that for me, neither compromise nor picking a single path is possible, and that instead of compromise or choice I must find a way for these beings to coexist, to live in synthesis or symbiosis. I don't know what that means, exactly, but it feels right.

It occurs to me now that this creature, which seemed even at the time of my near-death experience to be a man-boy, is neither boy nor man but both: the spirit of the boy I was born as and the spirit of the old man I will live to be, if I am lucky. Like the Watcher, he is always there, looking at what is going on in various corners of my being. Unlike the Watcher, he is allowed to intervene, and perhaps between us we can both find our way. Together, I think we can live a life, and when it comes time to die again, we will be ready.

Near-death is not a panacea and it comes with no guarantees, but it is an opening. Having been through much of my life a second time, I find some things have changed for the better: I have forgiven my mother, and she and I have started to become close; I am more solidly committed to writing; and I have begun, finally, to finish things I started 20 years ago. Others—my relationship with my father, for instance, and my inability to finally forgive him—have withstood both my near-death and his death unchanged, at least so far.

In the end, I'm not sure what it all means or if it means anything, really. One thing I know is that coming that close to death makes you aware of choices you didn't know you had before. And they are not small choices; they are all the choices there are. To borrow a phrase from science fiction, it is as if all the parallel universes in which you could have lived open up before you, as if they were all equally possible and equally likely. The weird thing is, they are. And the weirder thing is, they always have been, though it is only when you come out of a space in which there are no choices, there is only the waiting, that this multitude of possibility seems clear.

I don't know what the future will bring.

But then, nobody else does, either.

CRITICAL-THINKING ACTIVITIES

1. Explain in your own words exactly why it is that David Gordon performs a combined memorial service and birthday celebration each January 19th. Do his actions surprise you? Discuss your reaction.

2. How do you understand the events that led up to the near fatal hemmorhage? Would you have listened to Gordon when he attempted to resist the laxative preparation for the diagnositc test? What is your usual reaction when patients refuse prediagnostic preparations and other medications prescribed for them? Describe your philosophy for such situations.

3. What is the action of any laxative medication? Was the author correct in his thinking that the laxative would irritate his already bleeding bowel? Do you think that the diagnostic procedure should have been delayed?

4. What were your reactions to the author's story of the moment in time when he entered another space, leaving the hospital room? Discuss this event in relation to the beliefs of the Tibetan Buddhists the author mentions.

5. Do you have any quarrel with the words of the surgical resident that "they [doctors] intentionally give surgical patients drugs which not only relax but also erase short-term memory, so that they will forget anything they hear or feel while they are under anesthesia?" Discuss your response in detail and describe the policy of your surgical department. Do you see any ethical problems with this practice?

6. Given the information in this narrative, how would you have conducted the surgical procedure?

7. The author's brother visited him in the ICU and noted that David was never quite sleeping but seemed hypervigilant. His eyes would snap open during conversation and he looked as if he were in complete terror. What do you think was happening to the author during that time that would lead to such a response? Elaborate.

8. Do you feel it is appropriate to discuss with patients how their postsurgical pain will be managed? What factors should be part of this conversation? How would you assure the patient that the plan would be adhered to even in your absence? Be practical as well as theoretical in your answer.

9. How has the author's traumatic experience at Sister's Hospital and the aftermath affected his sense of himself and his relation to health-care professionals? Discuss in detail, giving examples from the narrative.

10. How has the author been able to integrate what happened to him for now and for his future? Elaborate with examples and discuss each.

Jean Pélégri

Jean Pélégri, born in Algeria and a longtime resident of Paris, is author of novels, plays, and essays. Among his many writings the most famous are the prize-winning novels *Les Oliviers de la justice* and *Le Maboul*. The first of these was made into a film by American filmmaker James Blue.

In addition, he has played character roles in several films, including *Pickpocket* by Robert Bresson, *Thérèse* by Alain Cavalier, *The Grand Carnival* by Alexandré Arcady, and *Fréquence Muerte* by Elisabeth Rappaneau, playing with Catherine Deneuve, to mention a few.

Jean Pélégri suffered an angina attack in his Paris home 3 weeks after the Gulf War began. Here he portrays his vivid recollections of the phantasmic episodes he experienced when he was thought to be in a coma owing to a miscalculation of an anesthesiologist during a coronary bypass procedure.

CHAPTER 10

The Strange Voyage*

by Jean Pélégri

What is most admirable in the fantasy world is that the fantasy does not exist, everything is real.

André Breton

*I*t was 1991. Three weeks before the Gulf War broke out, radios and televisions were talking about Operation Desert Storm, "furtive" planes, Scuds, severe war, and Soviet tanks maneuvering in Latvia. And in early February, as if I had participated in this war, I was driven to the hospital. Stretched out in an ambulance, it was the first time I saw Paris reduced to the top floors of its buildings.

I suffered from angina. After a few days of tests it was decided that I would undergo a triple bypass. The evening of the operation, the surgeon paid me a visit and reassured me that this operation was routine. As I listened on my portable radio to the reports of the American troops approaching Kuwait, the nurses prepared me for the next day's operation. They carefully shaved my chest and I found myself back in my bed with the hairless body of an adolescent.

When I woke up from the operation, I took back my little radio and I learned, with much amazement, that the French troops were approaching Baghdad and that they had crossed the desert in one day. *They are terrific, those French*, I thought to myself. What I did not know is that toward the end of my operation my heart had begun to fibrillate, and as a precaution, the surgeon had closed everything up and put me under deeper anesthesia.

Without my being aware of it, this anesthesia lasted 10 days and the strange voyage began. I was able, upon awakening, to recover some images of this voyage, sometimes complete and sufficient and sometimes made of deformed bits and pieces, like the paintings of Braque or Picasso. I sometimes had the impression of circulating within myself in some sort of museum of modern art, and of disposing of a cubistic memory. On the other hand, since they had strapped me to my bed so that I would not reopen my wounds, I often saw myself sleeping Christ-like, as on a cross.

---

*Translated from the French "L'Etrange Voyage," by Sameera Atallah.

Most important, because I was anesthetized for 10 days, it was impossible for me to conform my illusions to reality as I do in ordinary life. Despite this disorder and the lack of clear referents, and while everything was either imaginary or residing in the unconscious, I did maintain a sense of presence and coherence so strong that I could relate this voyage in a realistic way.

Everything was concrete and tangible and was inscribed in my mind with the certitude of the present.

This strange voyage is characterized by a succession of places or houses and by the reassuring presence of Serge, my Martiniquean nurse, and by Karim, a young but relentless nurse who took pleasure in giving me all sorts of injections at every opportunity.

The first house is situated in a forest, not too far from some sort of inn with closed window shutters. It's nighttime, it's raining in a steady stream, and a few hundred meters away beyond a curtain of trees, beams of crossed headlights indicate the presence of a highway. I'm stretched out in the window of a large antique shop, which is furnished haphazardly, with a small empty stage in the back. As for me, strapped to my bed, under the watchful gaze of Serge, I don't have the right to move.

Next, I am in a large country house. I am still forbidden to get up, but I have a vague memory of having written a book in this residence: a very engaging and militant piece that I could read on the walls and in my own handwriting, old pompous arguments. . . . And without any transition I find myself in a little village in the United States in an empty self-service place that belonged, like the rest of the village, to a rich "philanthropic pioneer" (like Philip Morris?). I am attached and cramped on some sort of metallic carriage in the midst of counters loaded with different articles, and I try to free myself in vain.

Another time, I stay on the outskirts of a village, at the edge (or the other side) of the Spanish frontier, in a narrow room where, as in the self-service place, I am stretched out on a very short slab. My feet extend onto a bedside table full of capsules and medications—and repeatedly, despite my protests, I undergo the torture of blood-letting by clumsy and pitiless Karim. . . . A question keeps coming up, constantly and obsessively: *Is it the afternoon—or is it already tomorrow*? I have to be taken to an inn in the neighborhood before I am brought back to Bichat, my Parisian hospital. And in anticipation, as it is getting dark outside, I hear the ambulance arriving. Before it happens, I see the door open and the medics enter, and I see them installing me on a stretcher. Suddenly they go out again, leaving me alone on the stretcher, asking myself, *When will I see my wife and son again*?

Here I am now lying on a mobile stretcher in a theater between rows of empty seats. The curtains don't open, I just wait for no reason. Like Godot. Maybe Serge, my nurse, looks for me in the little street that leads to the theater? I manage to detach myself, but it is impossible to run away.

Always the anguished need to warn the surgeon, through my nurse Serge, to make contact with my people. But I'm not sure that he has understood me.

(Here an empty interval without any images. What follows is of a different order.)

Serge, my nurse, brings me into the basement of the hospital for examination. I am on some sort of a theater stage, stretched on my mobile slab, and Serge is right next to me. At the end of the empty room, abstract paintings are rotating around an ax, and I wonder what could this exam be for. Soon, the voices of two women reach me from behind these paintings, and I try to understand what they are saying. Suddenly, one says, *I think this is the moment to get rid of him*! And the other agrees. Since I am tied down and it is impossible for me to defend myself, this menace frightens me, and I warn Serge about it. *Why do they want to kill me*? Finally, by listening hard, I am able to understand the strange reasoning that compels them to get rid of me. I am actually presumed to be in possession of a rare manuscript by Goethe (!) and they want to get hold of it. What amazes me is that this manuscript is by Goethe. I have many times attempted to understand his work, but in vain because of the inadequacy of translations or the incompatibility of languages; the same with Pushkin. Therefore, why would I have a rare manuscript by such a renowned writer? The question remains unanswered.

Next I am under a cloudy sky, on the shore of a vast lake, like the Bay of Algiers. There is a high building, white, functional, with glass windows instead of walls. . . . I am in the entrance, alone and abandoned on an infirmary's rolling stretcher. I wait; then I try to come down off my stretcher. A voice, somewhere, informs me that they are finally going to operate on me for a clot in my right leg. A nurse comes to get me and pushes my stretcher through a maze of gray hallways. I am very cold. We arrive at a large operating theater without any windows and with the metallic walls of a warship (without doubt, a cruiser). The surgeon is unknown to me, but I appeal to him to warn my people. *I am a prisoner*!

Suddenly, I am in the middle of a desert, attached to a luggage rack on the roof of a Volkswagen. My arms are stretched out as if on a cross. (Maybe this is where I think of Christ for the first time.) I make desperate attempts to detach myself, but the dreaded Karim arrives, assisted by a black American female nurse. *Well done, Mr. Pélégri. Now you can no longer move*, she says. And while she punctures my arm with her syringe, I see, far away, as if it is a mirage, the image of an Iraqi tank destroyed by an artillery shell and abandoned in the sand. I tell myself, *This shell is me*!

(*The decor changes. Maybe I left the recovery room for a stark room where I am alone?*)

■

As a starting and focal point, my room is a place fitted halfway with windows (which I do not actually discover until later upon waking), and beyond those windows are other successive stark rooms. In one of them, a man writes with an old pen on a small table. Behind him is a robot dressed in 18th-century style. The robot is holding a violin and repeats the same semicircular gesture tirelessly with its bow, in a muted way. From this I derive a very strong feeling of anxiety. By association, the man who is writing seems to be a robot himself, and I, in this world of absences, I am also not far from that state. Only the pain reminds me that, though remote, I am alive. On the right, behind several thick panes of glass, there are two other robots in profile: two greyhounds with sharp snouts, who, fixated on the journey, advance and retreat in a slow, mechanical, and ceaselessly repeated motion.

Always the same double windows. One startling day, in a different stark room, many people in white blouses followed by a rolling stretcher transport someone covered with a white sheet. They seem to have returned from an operation that he had missed; most of them, especially the youngest, seem exhausted. Only the chief surgeon, short and heavy, is very satisfied with himself, and with a forced laugh tells several medical jokes that nobody seems to be interested in.

Later, for one or two days, with other nurses, they transport me into other rooms and beyond, into other remote houses. I have no memory of the trip, only a feeling of solitude that grows as each day passes. First, a small apartment without windows, stocked with antique furniture (sofa, tapestry). Next, in the suburbs, a group of buildings without any character. Then, on the ground level of a large building a studio that belongs to one of the nurses. And always this tormenting question: *Is it afternoon—or already tomorrow?* It is no doubt the afternoon. Then, not very far from Bichat, a large bourgeois apartment, cold and anonymous, on Nouveau Boulevard—and always the same nurse with her syringe. I want to telephone my home, but I no longer know my number. I search for it patiently and painfully for hours—but in vain. The same the following days.

Another change of decor: a large room with white walls, in a Moorish style, with a painting drawn by a Tunisian and about which I was sure I wrote an article in the *Nouvel Observateur* (directed by Jean Daniel, my high school friend at the Lycée d'Algérie). With this came many childhood images: I am in a native Algerian farmhouse and I receive a phone call from Blida. It is Jean Daniel: He warns me that some strange person just took one of the red Blida buses. I hurry to the main highway on a pogo stick to catch up—but I wait in vain. The red car goes by without stopping.

(*Since seeing the painting by the Tunisian painter, I seem to be reunited, not by a reality that I had lived, but by an imaginary and dreamlike state that once seized me.*)

■

I return to the Moorish room: Paris is beneath the window, I know it—*but in what district?* And all of a sudden, one morning, in my room, it is Africa! A large black sun goddess in a provocative blouse—shiny jet-black, imposing, superb, with a dazzling smile. From what I understood, she takes care of the sanitary material. With her, nothing could go wrong, and around her everyone smiles. Then without any sound another black nurse arrives, older, with an emaciated, wrinkled face, in a copper-colored uniform. She resembles an old Indian woman, and immediately, as if I have known her in another life, I recognize her name: *Bois de Campêche*. Those two black women brought me peace. The first with her sunny shine, the second because, leaning over me, she touches me with her finger on the chest, the neck, the shoulders, while murmuring some sort of magical formulas. With them, and through them, I felt good: *Africa protects me!*

■

I am with Serge, the male nurse, always stretched on my rolling slab. I am in a vast basement at Bichat, with a very high ceiling, partitioned with glass panels, behind which all sorts of medical materials are arranged. Serge disinfects everything. At a lower level, and behind one of these glazed partitions, my anesthetist explains with great precision his techniques of anesthesia to a young nonresident student: *Do not insert very much. Use weak doses, but in a refined form.* With a sign of my thumb I make him understand that I appreciate his short speech very much. He responds with a smile.

■

Finally, finally, my people—my wife, my son—*dressed in blue and masked with blue, like some Tuaregs!* They announce that I will leave the recovery center and return to the room in Bichat where I had come from. I still have the power of joy! Then I'm informed there will be a period of convalescence (maybe in the south?).

■

Returning and waking up in my first room, I recover a sense of reality, but this reality seems to me unreal and contaminated: through the window, 10 floors below, the highway is filled with care—I have a vision of the end of the world with a grand temple in the style of the Pantheon or of the White House.

Sleep, waking, what time is it, what day? A narcissistic need to take refuge in my bed, in my dreams. Feelings of the vanity of the whole thing, and even, sometimes, the regret of not having died during the operation. A sentence by Bernanos seizes and imprisons me: *At the moment of death we enter the substance of being.* And posed on a shelf, next to the ceiling, images from the television; unbelievably artificial, exhausting, repetitive. All of these personalities who pass by seem to me like robots, and everything like mere publicity—even a football game. I prefer listening to the radio. *The French troops are close to Baghdad.* My wife, who comes every day from the other side of Paris, seems to me more and more exhausted. And Michel, my son, comes every night at dinner time. It is the first time that we have had such intimate conversations.

The friends, the visitors. It seems that the war is over.

Five months later, around the end of August, at Gault-la-Forêt, I plant dahlia bulbs; they are 3 months late and have already started to germinate in their carton. The stems are long, anemic, whitish—like me coming out of the hospital—but after a week and despite the delay, the stems have hardened, and turned purple; soon, the leaves have grown, and then the first blooms—and never have the dahlias been so beautiful!

Illness has taught me that nature works on us of itself and on its own terms.

CRITICAL-THINKING ACTIVITIES

1. How are the correspondences between historical and personal events manifested in Jean Pélégri's unconscious state?

2. As a writer and teacher the author has a deep appreciation for literature and art. How has this appreciation and knowledge converged with his treatment and subsequent fears?

3. Are you surprised by the fact that the author sensed that he was being moved from the ICU to other areas of the hospital and has misinterpreted the intentions of his nurses and other caretakers? How would you apply this knowledge when caring for a patient in similar circumstances?

4. It seems that the author has some recollection of the moment of induction to a deeper state of anesthesia. How has he interpreted this moment?

5. The author's experience of being transported by vehicles and stretchers and lying in bed vulnerable to others has a frightening quality. How would you have comforted him during those moments even though he was probably unconscious?

6. How would you interpret Pélégri's words, "Illness has taught me that nature works on us of itself and on its own terms?"

7. How many levels does the author show us that the human mind can function on at any given moment? Discuss fully.

Eugene Higgins

Eugene Higgins earned a BA and an MA from Harvard University. He is author of fiction and essays and teaches English literature and English as a second language at Dade Community College in Miami, the largest community college in the United States. He has lived and taught extensively in France, Spain, and Turkey.

In a period of 3 months, after turning 65, he underwent three surgical procedures and was discharged prematurely from the hospital without appropriate or even elemental home care in place. Here he shares the consequences and provides guidelines for humane care.

CHAPTER 11

Get 'Em out of the Shed

by Gene Higgins

Last summer I turned 65. A couple of months later my body began to fall apart like an overaged automobile, as if on command from social security.

In a period of 4 months, I had three operations—all different. What I learned from these several procedures is that hospitals are very anxious to get your money—or your insurance (may God have mercy on anyone without coverage)—and to get you out of the shed as fast as possible.

After major prostate surgery, I was out in 2 1/2 days. Because of the advanced state of a large cancerous tumor on my left leg between the knee and the ankle, I found myself back in the hospital a few weeks after the "TURP" (transurethral resection of the prostate), or as one nurse put it, the Roto-rooter. The leg was in bad shape, and it took a 2-inch by 3-inch skin graft from my thigh to cover the rather broad and deep wound.

I was supposed to go home the same day after that operation. But the surgeon had a problem with a patient at another hospital and arrived 5 hours late, which meant I had to spend those 5 plus hours in the busy pre-op room, or whatever they call it. It's the kind of place where a brief stopover is enough. And when the doctor arrived, late in the afternoon, he said he would arrange for me to stay overnight since it was late. A nurse then came in and doctored my IV, and in a few minutes I was off into a la-la land of overhead bulbs, new faces, green uniforms, masks, motion, and the rest of it. I didn't remember having dinner; I do remember not wanting to have breakfast.

After the doctor's perfunctory morning visit, he told me I could go home. He also informed me that I had a cast on my left leg to immobilize my ankle, which meant no walking on the foot.

I pondered that. My apartment is up one flight—no elevator. I live alone; my kids are away working or at college. The crash release program went into gear after the insurance company was contacted, naturally, and I was in a wheelchair for a quick lesson in walking on crutches. I was still weak, unsteady, and at age 65, not exactly as adept as I had been when I played three sports.

The crutch lesson was a flop. I was clearly too out of balance to do it. On came a walker; this, though easier, was still a drag, and I could not avoid putting weight on my just-operated-upon foot and leg. Given a choice, I selected the walker.

An hour later I was dressed and ready to go. Two Spanish-speaking men, armed with my name and address, came with a collapsible wheelchair. I was signed out, and the next thing I knew I was in an ambulette—a vanlike vehicle.

Between my room in the hospital and the van not a word of English passed their lips. This is a fact of life here in Miami where half of the population speaks Spanish. Still, I would like to have heard a sprinkling of words in my native tongue. I gave up on that, and since I know some Spanish, having lived in Spain for half a year, I directed them in their own language. It still took twice as long as usual to manage the mere 3 miles to my apartment.

Then came the dialogue in the parking lot while strategy was discussed as to how to get me from floor 1 to floor 2. Clearly, these two guys were not happy about that, just as I was getting fed up hearing them rattle on in a foreign language. Hell, when I was in their country and the others I lived in, I learned their language and I was *not* planning to stay there forever.

They got me to the top of the stairs, rolled me to the door, and then I was home and they were gone.

Home care went into operation after a hiatus of 3 days because it was a weekend. First, crutches were delivered because the walker I had was useless. Then, 2 days later, a male nurse came to teach me how to use the crutches—which were too small. New ones had to be ordered. Meanwhile, I had to get to the doctor for a dressing change, so I used the walker and a friend drove me.

The doctor said I should have nursing care to change the dressings, but it had to be arranged through the insurance company. Meanwhile, larger crutches arrived and the incorrect ones were removed. I was given a crash course by the male nurse in how to propel myself, especially up and down the steep stairway. I never did have enough strength to manage the crutches, but at least some of the weight was removed from the healing limb.

The dressing care kicked in a few days later. Each time it was a different nurse: the first was from the Bahamas, the second from Nigeria, and number three was from Miami. They meant well, but only one of them put on a dressing that did not start to unravel 3 hours after the application. So I informed the doctor that I could change the dressing myself, having seen it done enough times.

Observations: each and every time something is to be done, it has to be cleared through channels. Also, I always got the feeling, at least that was what came through to me, that there is an overwhelming rush to get you in and out. I was glad to be out, but I faced difficulties there because of the foul-up of time and a signed piece of paper. For that reason, I am glad to have had a couple of close friends who shopped for me and did things I could not do. Without them, I would have been utterly at sea. So I dedicate this to my true home care people, my friends Sonya, Peggy, and David. They brought the real help I needed and never let me down.

After the third surgery, on a hernia—as I said, it wasn't my year—I was supposed to once again leave the hospital on the same day, but since the doctor was delayed, I stayed overnight.

Many of the people I met in the course of my peripatetic journey down pain alley, not to mention home care, were efficient enough, I suppose. I didn't die or go into convulsions. But a warm human touch was missing. For the most part I felt like meat. In the recovery room after my first surgery, I rambled on to one nurse's aide, who kept saying yes to all my questions—which happened to center on books. Even in my semidrugged, loose-tongued "dream bloom," I realized that she probably had not read all the books that I reeled off. I think she was humoring me, or being defensive, or both.

Actually, the best nurse I had was deaf. As soon as she spoke to me I could tell. But she told me anyway. She was genuinely warm. We discussed our families and her deafness. She was sincere in her concern, truly compassionate, and caring, simply because she was direct and had her own problems.

That, I think, unites those who share this planet. Suffering is everywhere, and when one has passed through that cauldron, a sincere hand and heart survive in the mind as the warmest of memories. Be interested in people, their lives and their families. It is vital that you not feel like a total patient. Hell, we're all patients in this universe we share now.

CRITICAL-THINKING ACTIVITIES

1. Discuss the examples from this account that show us why Gene Higgins felt like meat rather than a human being during and after the three hospitalizations.

2. What would have made his three experiences with the health-care system reasonable? Design a plan for conducting his care through the surgical procedures, postoperative period, and home care.

3. Why is it upsetting for someone who is ill not to be able to speak and communicate clearly and freely with his or her caretakers. How would you manage such a reality if you were the hospital administrator?

4. What is inappropriate about the nurse's explanation of the TURP? Take into consideration her phrase and its potential effects on a vulnerable patient.

5. Elaborate on the author's premise that it is important to individuals who become ill not to feel that they are merely patients, and nothing more.

6. This author reminds us that we are all patients in the universe we share. How does this affect the way you view yourself as a health-care professional?

James Armstrong

James Armstrong earned a BA and an MA in English literature from Penn State University and served in the United States Army. He teaches English literature and composition in a public high school in Philadelphia.

His father was diagnosed with Parkinson's disease 7 years ago and subsequently developed chronic, episodic, and at times severe lower abdominal pain. Despite countless diagnostic procedures and hospitalizations, the origin of this pain has never been discovered. What emerges in this account is a mystifying unhappiness factor for his father and mother that is elusive and unsolvable by the primary practitioners and specialists.

CHAPTER 12

An Unhappiness Factor

by James Armstrong

My father's illness was first diagnosed approximately 7 years ago. We weren't given a whole lot of information or preparation for what would follow. Generally speaking, the physician merely said the tremors would get worse—he had Parkinson's disease. There may have been more information, but this was the best my mother could relate at the time. I am reasonably sure that she was accurate 7 years ago.

Shortly thereafter, things changed. My father experienced dramatic bouts of pain—a severe burning in the lower pelvic area and groin. This resulted in several emergency room visits over the next year. Sometimes he spent 3 or 4 days in the hospital. All the usual tests were done, and occasionally some minor infection would be found, but nothing was ever identified as the actual cause of the pain.

The next year things picked up: emergency room visits, doctor's appointments, urologists, and so forth. My parents, who had been living in West Virginia until my father retired as a plant manager, decided to move home to be closer to friends and local doctors and, of course, me. Soon we had gone from seeing doctors every 2 or 3 months to almost every month. This included trips to the emergency room at any time of night and two or three visits to the family doctor and urologist in the same month. There were a lot of visits and a lot of doctors and one lengthy stay at the Hospital of the University of Pennsylvania. I wasn't there for all the visits, but my involvement had increased considerably.

There was always one big mystery: What was the cause of the intense pain and why didn't my dad show any visible reaction to it? I can still see the faces of the doctors; they would look at my dad and then at me, as if to say, "What's up? Why doesn't he react?" Then they would prescribe a pain killer and send him home or, occasionally, to a hospital for more tests. He had every pain killer in the book, including morphine. It was their way of taking care of the problem. This only increased, as time passed. Sometimes I would see his discomfort at home; but it was never evident to doctors. By now he had seen every doctor in town and nothing had changed.

He was wasting away during all of this. He got physically smaller and smaller. Mother had him on a low-fat diet—wrong! She had also picked up some new skills. She was catheterizing him and giving him enemas way beyond what was necessary (not to mention that she shouldn't have done any of it). Furthermore, none of the doctors saw that she was getting forgetful.

From there we went to adult foster care, which lasted only a few months. Then we went to nonskilled care and then to skilled nursing care.

At first I thought I would be relieved. However, with my parents now separated, my father in a nursing home and my mother in an apartment, the worst months of my life began. I was completely stressed out waiting for something bad to happen to both. I couldn't stand the telephone. I would jump out of my skin when it rang, and I would wake up in the middle of the night *thinking* I heard the phone.

Eventually, something bad *did* happen. One night my father began having seizures. So it was back to the ER, the hospital, and the doctors. The first year and a half was hell because he wasn't happy, he threatened to "do something" to himself, and he kept calling relatives and asking them to "come and take me from the home." This was a terrible time; I didn't want to see him; however, I did, two or three times a week. I had trouble sleeping, I was irritable, and I felt trapped. I still jumped at a ringing phone no matter where I was. I dreaded going home and looking at the answering machine. I was jealous of my sister's freedom (she doesn't live in the United States) and I felt totally trapped. It was as if all my plans and dreams were over just because I had made the mistake of staying in my home town while my parents had followed my dad's work elsewhere. On top of this, I felt guilty because I love my parents and I felt terrible about what was happening to my father.

My only relief has been the nursing home because at least he has nurses and aides around him. He is safe and I am not on call 24 hours a day. I can breathe for the first time. I can go to work and come home to a somewhat normal life. I still feel as if I am in a trap, but I can function now. Until you are the person that is in charge of everything you will never fully understand.

There are still battles with social workers and Medicaid. I won't tell about the months of hell that caused. Then there are the social workers who fail to look at the entire problem, and therefore they create new ones when they try to take him out of skilled care. It is a never-ending circle. You feel like nobody will help because everybody causes problems. This isn't entirely true, but it feels this way most of the time. Meanwhile I can now relate to my family and even the people I work with. That is, until the next problem shows up.

What does cause the pain? Is it spasmodic bladder, as one urologist thinks? Is it a bladder infection, as many doctors thought? One out of four times there might be one, but after all of the trips to the ER and all of the office visits, this was all they could ever come up with. That's over 7 years, three hospitals, seven or eight specialists, and probably 20 doctors. This is it! Not much of an answer. Mother clings to the experts. She can't handle the possibility that it might be emotional distress—or what I call an unhappiness factor. She always grasps at some thread of information from a past doctor. In fact, many times she encouraged the doctor appointments.

What really happened to my father when he realized he had Parkinson's? What effect did this have on both my parents? When it happened, they lived alone and out of town. I know they stressed each other terribly after my dad's retirement, but I can't be diagnostically positive. Nevertheless, consider the following:

- They isolated themselves and spent a lot of time together. Could this have created some resentment on both their parts?

- They have a history of getting on each other's nerves. My mother was especially good at this. She could pick and pick until my dad reacted.

- At the beginning, as at the end, the doctors didn't provide any answers. Did Dad create situations to get help from the doctors?

- Did he do it to make my mother jump or be more sympathetic?

■ Is it a combination of these things: Parkinson's plus caustic relationship plus resentment plus age-related physical problems?

Whatever it is, it is perplexing.

I know he got through the pain situations without the ER and medications at foster care, in the hospital (where they used placebos), and at home. Very seldom did one see any actual indication of suffering. The next day he would relate how bad it was and appear much better. But if asked if he was better, he would say, "No! I still have it!" He would snap at my mother when she asked. He wouldn't argue with me, except when he thought I might be doubting him.

I think Dr. Davis's placebo injection plan was the only time a doctor explored the possibility of an emotional cause. This could account for some of the lack of attention by both of the local doctors. They would treat the physical and throw up their hands at the emotional.

Finally, I don't think anyone has an answer. It is as if it is too new or an unexplored area. Is it an emotional problem brought on by disease, resentment, the end of the marriage in real sharing terms, or simply the inability to deal with all of these things?

I don't know the answer and neither do the doctors thus far. However, they should try to recognize the unhappiness factor and understand its effect on one's physical and emotional state.

CRITICAL-THINKING ACTIVITIES

1. What are some of the causes of intermittent chronic pain? Do individuals suffering from chronic pain usually appear to be suffering? If not, why? Discuss.

2. Do you think that this family received appropriate counseling and guidance when Parkinson's disease was diagnosed? Elaborate.

3. Is pain an integral part of Parkinson's symptomatology? Explore this concept in the current scientific literature.

4. What are placebos? How are they utilized? When are they legitimate and worth-while?

5. How is the unhappiness factor manifested in this narrative?

6. Devise a model of care for this family, taking into consideration each member's separate needs and responsibilities.

7. As the primary practitioner for this family, what would alarm you regarding the increasingly frequent and essentially uneventful (though painful and invasive tests and examinations) experienced by Mr. Armstrong?

8. The author of this account has experienced long-term stress from the nearly 7 years of attempting to assist his parents. What are your concerns for his health and welfare? His family's?

9. James Armstrong's parents were eventually separated. How do you imagine this affected their emotional states after more than 60 years of married life together? Discuss, using examples from the account and knowledge about attachment and loss and social and cultural expectations.

10. Exactly how would you humanize Mr. Armstrong's care and way of life? Elaborate fully.

11. Is there an unhappiness factor that causes pain and painlike symptoms that is beyond the competence of medical experts but nevertheless causes real "holistic" suffering? Could this suffering be similar to that of fear and sorrow?

Mark Maclean Rufo

Mark Maclean Rufo earned his JD at Boston University School of Law and his BA in the College of Liberal Arts at Boston University. He lives in Nashua, New Hampshire, where he specializes in personal-injury law.

Here Rufo describes his work with and for a 19-year-old young man permanently disabled in a diving accident. He argues for the community's institutions and the legal system's support for this young man so that he can live safely and decently.

CHAPTER 13

Get the Money

by Mark Maclean Rufo

I am a trial lawyer for physically injured plaintiffs. I first heard of Sean Michael Garrity through a phone call from his father. I have no idea how he got my name.

Before hearing the tale, you should know something about how my business works. I deal with misery. I don't cause it. I don't buy it or sell it. I am only a middleman. If you can keep that in mind, what follows will make sense.

Most of my cases begin with a phone call. (Occasionally someone drops by unannounced. But I don't see them. This isn't a barber shop, as I tell my secretaries.) Someone calls with a new case. Is it about an injury? Yes. Who was injured? Me, my wife, my husband, my boyfriend, my girlfriend, my son, my daughter—whatever. And *how* injured are you, your wife, your husband? This is where we separate the wheat from the chaff. The stubbed toes, the hurt feelings, the "but I was almost killed!" Chaff. Get rid of it.

Sean's injuries were not chaff. He was 19 years old and in the intensive care unit with a crushed cervical fifth vertebra and paralysis from the neck down. This was wheat, as in bread, as in dough. But I jump ahead. Zillion-dollar cases are everywhere. Like virtual particles in subatomic physics, they last slightly longer than a billionth of a second.

We have the damages. How about insurance? (After all, I do business in the United States, not the Land of Oz.) Sean was injured on the common grounds of a condominium complex. They have insurance up the wazzoo.

So far, so good. Two cherries have come up on the slot machine. But that third tumbler is still spinning. The liability tumbler. Please, please, please, make it easy. Tell me Sean was injured when he fell through a defective railing that the condo management knew all about but had not gotten around to fixing.

No such luck. Sean broke his neck diving into a swimming pool *from the shallow end*. I am going to have to earn the money on this one.

I go to see my client. Sean is in the hospital room, all wired up. I turn on the bedside manner. It isn't hard. I *do* feel sorry for him. He is 19 years old and will never walk again. Before his injury, health and youth were the only things Sean had going for him. He is a high school dropout. A manual laborer. His parents divorced when he was still a child. His upbringing was less than idyllic. But Sean had just started to acquire skills in the construction trade when he had his unfortunate encounter with the concrete bottom of the swimming pool.

At this point, Sean is still in that early stage that I see so often, and that separates the big injuries from the little injuries like a continental divide. With the little injuries, people exaggerate at first. But with the big injuries, it is always the other way around. It takes quite a while for things to sink in. First comes the sheer gratitude at being alive. Then the feeling that with so many people *trying* to make you feel better, you must be a bum if you don't tell them that they are succeeding. Then comes the let's-take-it-one-step-at-a-time phase. Only later do they get to the dread handwriting-on-the-wall phase. (Just read nurses' and physical therapists' notes. The whole progression is there.)

I get the basic facts of the accident. But these are a bit fuzzy. Again, this is a divide between big injuries and little injuries. With the little injuries, the clients tend to prattle on like morons and give all kinds of superfluous detail. With the big injuries, it is like pulling teeth to find out what happened.

From Sean, I can get only a bare-bones account. He was cold sober when he dove into the pool. (My first concern, and the medical records bear him out.) He and his friends were just cooling off on a hot afternoon. Everyone having a wonderful time, right up until. . . .

The diving from the shallow end is still going to be a problem. But when God closes a door, he opens a tiny crack in the floorboards. The dimensions of the pool are such that it is actually hazardous to dive into *any* part of it. But a layperson would be easily fooled into thinking otherwise. (They even put blue liners on the damn things to give you the illusion of oceanic depth.) So is there any warning sign against diving into the pool? Well, yes—but the condominium management put it up *after* the accident.

We have a case.

I write some letters. The insurer for the condominium complex gets in touch with me. They say Sean caused his own injuries. Standard insurance company crap. They offer me $5000 to pay medical bills—but they have no choice about that. Sean was injured on the premises, so the med pay is due him automatically, regardless of fault. However, this actually presents the first crisis of the case.

I write to Sean and explain the situation. Yes, he has a case. But no, the insurance comply is not going to pay millions of dollars because they want to do good deeds. If a jury decides that Sean is more than 50 percent responsible for his own injuries, then nothing will be awarded, regardless of the extent of injury. A jury will almost certainly decide that Sean is responsible to some degree for diving into the shallow end of a swimming pool. Therefore, the case will be a long and difficult one, with the outcome impossible to predict.

That leaves the $5000 med pay. It can be swallowed up in the black maw of the health-care system. Or it can be put to good use financing the case, paying for medical records to be copied, the swimming pool expert who will be needed to testify for us at the trial, and the other out-of-pocket expenses that will have to be incurred. (Of course, five grand will not be enough for all this. I will have to foot the additional expenses myself. But $5000 is still $5000.)

After a slight delay, I hear back from Sean. He would like me to just mail him the $5000.

What the hell is he going to do with it in the hospital? Buy flowers for himself? But it is his money. I mail it to Sean, with a letter explaining that if he is not willing to make this investment into his own case, then I cannot help him. I wish him all the luck in the world, and add that he has 3 years from the date of injury in which to bring suit.

File closed. Story ended. For a while.

More than 2 years later, Sean calls me. He wants to know if he can still bring a lawsuit. He has never gotten any money other than the $5000 I sent him.

And what happened to the money? It seems that Sean's father read my letter and persuaded Sean that suing would be a waste of time. It was better, the father explained, to give *him* the $5000 so that he could use it for Sean's own good. Sean did this, and never saw one penny of the money again.

Daddy is now out of the picture.

The 2-year delay may have spared me possible headaches. Sean has come to grips with his condition as a quadriplegic. He has some limited use of his arms. He has mobility in a wheelchair. And he is living with Jean, a divorced woman who had been one of his therapists. They are quite happy together.

Something else I have noticed about the major injuries. The victim goes through a dark spell. But when he comes out of it, he shows a psychologically amazing acceptance of his condition and a reasonable desire to make the best of things. This is in sharp distinction to the minor-injury victim, who with the passage of time is *more* likely to whine about the injustice of life and how everyone has taken advantage of him.

I explain to Sean that the 3 years are not up. He can still bring a lawsuit. The condominium complex is still there. The insurance company is still doing business. And his case still has all the problems it had before.

But nothing ventured, nothing gained. We sue.

Two years and $10,000 dollars later. . . .

The case is about to go to jury trial. The insurer made an offer of $20,000 to settle when I first told them we were bringing suit. There have been no offers since. Everyone even remotely connected with the accident has been deposed. We have Sean's neurologist on videotape. We have a pool expert standing by to testify for us. We have an economist lined up to project future lost wages and medical expenses, discounted to present value. We have an RN and an LPN ready to testify for us. We have a bus scheduled to take the jury to see the pool.

Two weeks before the trial date, a "settlement conference" is held at the courthouse. This is a mandated procedure in which the two sides are supposed to attempt to arrive at a settlement in good faith. But to the vipers who run insurance companies, "good faith" is no more comprehensible than the fourth dimension or a new primary color. We go through the minor farce of the settlement conference with no offer of settlement at all.

None of the weaknesses of the case have disappeared. I know what I have to deal with. Sean knows it too, because I have told him. The odds are against us.

If it were only a question of Sean versus the mega-greed of the insurance company, then no jury would let Sean leave empty-handed. Unfortunately, my opponents always proceed through deception, and the political system supports them. A jury cannot be informed that a defendant has insurance. Therefore the illusion is created that any verdict in Sean's favor will have to be paid by the members of the condominium association directly. (This sensitivity to class hatreds is one of the dirty secrets of the American court system. Cases where a worker is trying to get compensation from the superrich are systematically misrepresented to juries as one working stiff trying to sock it to another working stiff.)

Curiously enough, my opponents' own propaganda can be turned to my advantage at this point. Insurers have spent millions of dollars deceiving the public into believing that plaintiffs with phony injuries and shyster lawyers are milking the system. But in the process, the insurers have also, albeit unintentionally, educated the public into the reality that nearly all business enterprises in the United States have private insurance. If Sean's case goes to trial, the jury will almost certainly realize that the condo association is insured to the hilt. And the jurors may prefer giving money to Sean than leaving it with a multizillion-dollar insurance company.

But how good is my reasoning? If my conclusion is the only logical one, then why has the insurer not reached the same conclusion and made a reasonable offer to settle the case? Or *have* they reached the same conclusion, but are waiting until the last minute to settle?

One week before trial, defense counsel tells me that the insurer wants a meeting. So the wall is cracking.

The day before the meeting, I am scheduled to fly to the Midwest to take the deposition of the other side's "pool expert." Should I waste a whole day on that foolishness, knowing that the case will likely be settled on the following day? I could ask to postpone the deposition. But no, that is not the way to do it. If I postpone, the other side will know I expect to settle the case at the meeting. That is why *they* have not asked to postpone the deposition. My opponents cut deep, but I cut deeper. I go ahead with the deposition and immolate a day to give the impression that I have no great hope of settling the case. Having done all this, I am now in the best position I can be to get my client the money.

Just prior to the conference, defense counsel inadvertently tips me off with a remark. "I can win this case 9 times out of 10!" he says. I do not say anything, but I think to myself, "You may be right, but you are telling me that you know you would lose this case 1 time out of 10. And how much would that cost your client?"

The conference is held at the courthouse, this being neutral ground. Sean and Jean are in the building, but in a separate room where I can speak with them privately. I walk back and forth, conveying an offer, countering with a demand, conveying a new offer, and so on. The insurer is being realistic now. But they didn't make all their money by being unrealistic.

And here is food for thought. At stake is, potentially, millions of dollars. The court system is ready to conduct a jury trial. Hundreds of hours of work have been put into the case on both sides. I don't know how many years of expertise are tied into it, if you include the lawyers, the insurance people, the pool experts, and the medical experts. And the final decision on whether to settle will be made by a high school dropout in a wheelchair.

But who else should decide? And here is another thing that separates the major injuries from the minor ones. The profoundly injured have a very clear vision of the possibilities open to them. They have an excellent grasp of reality. I do not believe that anyone's intelligence has ever been increased by a physical injury. But the profoundly injured are forced to apply their intelligence more efficiently. They will seek out good advice and follow it when they find it. They eschew fantasy, or neurotic dwelling on what might have been, or the polar idiocies of self-pity and false vengeance.

I can convey a settlement offer to my client. I can tell him what a reasonable response will be to keep negotiations going. I can tell him how far I think the insurers will go to settle. But the final decision on accepting settlement must be made by Sean.

But what does the insurance company get out of settling? This part is hard to explain, for it deals with what a jury *really* does. Read Canetti's *Crowds and Power*. A jury is a type of *increase pack*. So is a team of health providers. (Canetti does not use either example; he limits his discussion to primitive peoples, but the functions are the same.) An increase pack is a closed group engaged in rhythmic, stylized activities to bring about some increase in the prosperity of the tribe.

The Mandan Indians danced until the buffalo came. They said it always worked—because they would not stop dancing *until* the buffalo came. An increase pack is nearly always successful, in the eyes of its own members. The dance *must* go on until the objective is achieved. The jury must reach a verdict (mistrials are rare). Health providers always produce a favorable outcome by lessening the suffering of the patient (according to their own records—medical malpractice is another story for another time).

Dozens of people provided health services to Sean. Every one of them was convinced that the services were worthwhile. No one ever said, "Wouldn't he be better off dead?" Working individually, they might have thought this. Working as a pack, they did not have to. Their care was successful, not because they gave Sean a baclofen pump and a nice new wheelchair, but because they made *him* part of the increase pack. He was also dancing for the buffalo to come back.

Had the case gone to a jury, there were two possible outcomes. One is that the jurors would have seen Sean as an *outsider*, a person who engaged in a bizarre act that put him beyond the rest of us, so what does he expect us to do? He could even be seen as a threat. ("If I give him a lot of money, then my insurance rates will go up and I will be encouraging frivolous lawsuits!")

The other possibility was that Sean would be seen as *one of us*. He did something stupid and dangerous. But is jumping into the shallow end of a swimming pool any more stupid and dangerous than smoking cigarettes, not exercising, or overeating? If Sean is one of us, then we should find a way to help him. If we focus on the victim and not on where the money is coming from, then we want to go on doing our dance until the victim is made "well" and our own prosperity is thereby increased. This is what the insurance company is afraid of.

We get a good offer to settle. I push the insurance company to the limit of what they will pay to avoid a trial. Sean says to take it. I cannot gamble with other people's money. This case going to trial would have been a gamble, and the odds were against us. Instead, we beat the odds.

You will be spared the details of the relatives who showed up after the settlement and explained to Sean how they could handle this money for him. They did not get any of it. Even after the lien holders were paid, Sean received enough to buy a house, a handicap-equipped van, and then some. I still stay in touch with him. He and Jean are doing quite well. The insurance company avoided the risk for placing Sean's misery before a jury. They paid good money to avoid that. As for me, I got back the $10,000 I had invested in the case. And I got a day's pay.

As I said, I don't buy and sell misery. I am only a middleman.

CRITICAL-THINKING ACTIVITIES

1. Attorney Rufo states that he deals in misery, he doesn't cause it. Why is this crucial to our understanding for the profoundly injured?

2. How, then, is Rufo's business the same as or different from that of medicine?

3. Rufo implies that there are politics involved in the adversarial relationship between insurance companies and defense lawyers. How do you understand this political tension, and how might it affect this injured client's health and welfare?

4. What is your role in instances where a client has been profoundly injured? Would you support your client in a suit against the condominium owners? Why or why not? Defend your answer.

5. Is this author correct when he claims that at times insurance companies foster class hatreds? Have you ever seen an example of such behavior in health care? Discuss in detail.

6. Devise an investigative research project in which you explore the legal facts that health-care professionals should know in regard to the wrongfully injured.

7. Rufo tells us that he has gained his understanding, in part, of the progression from denial to acceptance of profound and permanently injured from nurses' and physical therapists' notes in the medical record. Were you aware that your assessments of a patient's emotional state could involve the scrutiny of the legal system and thus influence the patient's welfare long after discharge? Outline and discuss the way in which you assess an individual's emotional state with pristine accuracy.

8. Do you find yourself secretly blaming Sean for his accident? Why is this important for you to discover? How might this belief affect your attitude and behavior toward him?

9. Write a paper in which you discuss the responsibilities of developers and builders for their products and the safety of citizens who use them. Make links to all of the citizens in a community and their responsibility for one another.

Mark Nepo

Mark Nepo is a poet and philosopher who teaches at the State University of New York at Albany. His books include *God, the Maker of the Bed, and the Painter* (Greenfield Review Press, 1988), *Fire without Witness* (British American, 1988), and most recently, *Acre of Light* (Greenfield Review Press, 1994). He is presently completing two books of spiritual philosophy, *Rowing at the Pace of Clouds* and *While We Are Blossoms: The Journey beyond Selfing*. His essays appear regularly in *Voices, the Journal of the American Academy of Psychotherapists, Pilgrimage, the Journal of Psychotherapy and Personal Exploration*, and *Sufi*.

In 1987, Mark Nepo and his wife, Anne, were both diagnosed with cancer: and their world unraveled and had to be reordered. Their experience taught them to find the proper balance of self-will, prayer, and modern medicine in order to recover and to heal. Two poems, "Long-Term Care" and "The Music beneath the Music," elucidate and crystalize Nepo's experience of pain and emerging hope.

CHAPTER 14

God, Self, and Medicine

by Mark Nepo

Since long before the story of Job, human beings, the most fragile and durable of all the species, have had to deal with the paradox of suffering. And in our pain we ache to know how, if there is a God, can that eternal presence sanction pain and breakage, and further, in the face of all this, how can such an all-knowing force fuel us with the capacity and sensitivity to suffer so acutely. From the young slave crushed by a stone headed for the top of a pyramid to the senseless shooting of a clerk in Detroit, those left to grieve have asked in universal echo why, as the rest of us stand in silent chorus voicing a bewildered hymn that has lasted centuries.

It is no mistake that to suffer means *to feel keenly, to undergo, to experience.* And flexing our knot of blood that some call heart, we are blessed and cursed into the searing moments that both threaten and enrich our lives. For to feel keenly is the only path to transformation and wholeness, if it doesn't kill us first. And as with the stubborn rocks along the ocean, if we can endure the scouring, the pounding of the deep will in time reveal an inner beauty otherwise hidden. But we are not rocks. Our acuteness of perception and inner sensation, our unprecedented range of thought and mood, make us so vulnerable that we can die and be reborn daily; an emotional form of Prometheus. And so, our continual quest is to stay more renewed than devoured; our chief task, to find a way to gain enough from what is revealed to survive the pain of such opening.

That's the point of engaging our experience: to gain enough from what we feel to survive the pain in feeling it, to live through the thresholds that paradox offers, to live through the pain of breaking to the other side, into the rearrangement of nothing less than our very lives. And most importantly, we do not have to seek this sort of experience. We cannot avoid it. We have only to find the courage to internalize it.

This essay was originally put together from several books, published and in manuscript, for a dedication speech that was delivered on October 22, 1994, at the Fetzer Institute in Kalamazoo, Michigan, to celebrate the opening of the Institute's residential education center called Seasons: A Center for Renewal. It gave me the chance to coalesce much of where we've journeyed in the realm of mind, body, and spirit. Passages are drawn from *Acre of Light,* which recounts our experience with cancer and the transformation of our healing, as well as from two books of spiritual philosophy still in progress (*Rowing at the Pace of Clouds* and *While We Are Blossoms: The Journey beyond Selfing*). It also includes excerpts from my essay, "A Terrible Knowledge," which has been used as the thematic center of the 1994 issue of the Journal of Pastoral Counseling (Iona College).

My breaking has, indeed, led me into an expanding love of being that is clearly God. Both my wife and I have been broken by disease and know fully that there are moments endured from which our lives will never be the same; severe moments beyond which everything is changed. No one asks for these moments. They simply happen the way a merciless wind cracks a tree we never imagined would crack.

In 1987, my wife and I were both stricken with cancer. The months became a labyrinth. In May, Anne was diagnosed with cervical cancer. She had a conization in June and a hysterectomy in August. At the same time, a mysterious lump forming on my head turned out to be growing underneath the skull as well. It grew to the size of half a grapefruit. And so, mere days after her surgery, I entered the hospital, moving through a gauntlet of tests, including a biopsy that identified this strange lesion as a lymphoma lodged between my brain and skull. It was eating through the bone. Finally, after I experienced much desperation and prayer and visualization and fighting with and against doctors, the tumor, both below the skull and above, vanished; I avoided major brain surgery, whole-head radiation, and spinal chemotherapy.

The doctors could not explain it. Our friends and family helped us limp back to life, a struggle in itself, which we were shaping strongly until November 1988, when a spot on my eight rib began to grow. We were crushed. By January, the lump filled my wife's palm as we hugged. And in February 1989, I underwent thoracic surgery to remove that rib and its adjacent muscles. The cells in that rib had turned malignant, so, barely repaired, we embarked on 4 months of chemotherapy. Today, as of our last checkup, we are both well, and forever changed by this odyssey.

We have, quite frankly, found death at our shoulder earlier than most. Yet we have also been touched by a relentless, mysterious grace that has surfaced briefly to restore us. Repeatedly, it rises to save us or empower us—we can no longer make the distinction—and we find ourselves tied to a fathomless place where neither of us had dared to voyage. We call that reservoir God, though you may call it something else.

In truth, this experience has unraveled the way we see the world. It has scoured our lens of perception, landing us in a deeper sense of living. And though our story is framed around a particular crisis, cancer, we believe that crisis of the deepest kind somehow raises a common instinct to survive and with that a common set of tools becomes available to all. Having come this far, it seems clear that being a survivor is embracing the will to live, and that whether that embrace lasts for years or months or days or even hours, whoever embraces life is a survivor.

We were, against our will, reduced, with our mouths open, into the mystery of life in which we all swim and from which we all emerge to our separate shores. We know we were and are both weak and strong, stubborn and determined, afraid and brave, intrusive and demanding, resilient and stalled, confused and clear—sometimes all at once. We know now that going on without denying any aspect of the human drama is what strength is all about.

We know now that, being human, we are each the crucible, the ever-changing inlet through which the greater whole in all its forms ebbs and flows. Indeed, every time the universe, through nature or God, flows through us, we are rinsed larger, cleansed, and charged yet again. What is medicine, if not the laws of nature applied to cleanse the self. And what is God, if not the laws of spirit applied to enlarge the self. It implies that to enlarge is to cleanse; to grow is to heal. Thus, to talk about the art of healing is to investigate the various ways, both natural and spiritual, that the whole, if taken in, can preserve the part.

Initially, I felt a traumatic paralysis, the fast-breathing, huddled fear of a wounded animal lying still in the brush, expecting to be struck again. This is worse than outright pain, this is withdrawing from anything that can help. This is the power of fear—to make you recoil from anything larger. While in this state, nothing flows through and, therefore, nothing cleanses or enlarges. The center remains cut off when it needs to be renewed more than ever. And I believe how we first stand after doubling over is crucial to whether we will heal at all.

I was 36 when I was diagnosed with cancer, and up till then I had never been ill. I was terrified, and nothing was helping me conquer the fear. Finally, I was visited in a dream by the great Chinese poet of the Tang dynasty, Tu Fu.

> *Out of the yellow mist*
> *he came, his Oriental beard*
> *in tow. We were on a healthy shore*
> *and he sat cross-legged in the sand,*
> *scratching delicately with a branch,*
> *his slender head down. I crouched*
> *and put it to him, "How do I block*
> *the fear?" He kept scratching the sand*
> *as if he hadn't heard. I grew angry,*
> *"How do I block the fear?!" He lifted*
> *his head and shrugged,*
> *branch waving above him,*
> *"How does a tree*
> *block the wind?"*
> *With that, he*
> *disappeared.*

And so I was broken of my illusion that fear could be conquered. Instead, I began to watch the winter trees as they let the wind through, always through. And since, I have learned that fear gets its power from not-looking, that it is intensified by isolation, that it is always more strident when we are self-centered. Now, when I am full of fear, which can't be avoided, I try, though I don't always succeed, to break its stridency by breaking my egocentrism. I try to quiet its intensity by admitting my fear to loved ones, and I try to disempower its exaggeration by looking directly into exactly what I fear. I try to know that though I can be fearful, I am more than my fear.

But life under siege hides none of its difficulties. The endless decisions that must be made, each imperative and of great consequence, do not wait for us to manage our fear. Indeed, one is always *thrust* into the world of cancer and there is no escort. When my wife and I were so thrust, we uncannily met our counterparts, Janice and Tom. Janice was a strong, determined woman who believed primarily in self. She did not believe in medicine and therefore put her entire well-being and treatment into her own hands. She rejected all medical intervention, and if she used anything greater than her self, it remained a secret liaison till the end. She was tenacious but died a painfully drawn-out death. Now, there isn't a doctor's visit I don't feel Janice over my shoulder. I understand her resistance more and more, for the things we are asked to do to preserve our well-being are not pleasant. Yet in the hard breath before each decision, I see her reliance solely on self and fear its imbalance.

Tom, on the other hand, was adrift. He really had no sense of self and had a disinterested, entropic view of the world. He put his fate completely in the hands of medicine. And so, we watched Tom grow smaller in the space he took up. We watched Tom give no resistance whatsoever to what doctors wanted to do. Blake said, "Without contraries there is no progression."* Tom presented no healthy contrary, and thus there was no progression. He became invisible, vanishing piece by piece. By Christmas of that year, he no longer knew who we were. By February, he died.

I feel roughly blessed to have Tom and Janice as specters of where I must not go, though the further we travel here, the more compassion I have for how easily, in any given moment, the Tom or Janice in me can take over.

While Tom and Janice died, I was broken and healed and broken again. The first time, my tumor vanished. It was a miracle. When its sister began to thicken the rib in my back, I began with fervor the same rigorous visualizations and meditations and intensive prayers for hours each day, desperate to enlist the same overwhelming grace. But after 6 weeks, I was exhausted and humbled, for the tumor in my rib had only grown. I thought I had failed. The fear returned, now as terror. And in making my decision to have that rib removed, I heard Janice spurn my doctor and saw Tom with indifference bow. But I believe in God and in this strange familiar terrain called me, in which life and He meet. So, I waited 'til these elements merged, way down beneath my understanding, and there, in what felt like calm balance, I said yes, help me. With that, it became clear that this time, the *surgery* was the miracle.

Once home, it hurt so much to breathe that it took several tries to make it to my rocker where I moaned and thought, I have outlived a tumor pressing on my brain, and my eighth rib is gone, and though I'd wept in the tub at the gash in my side, at the fact that I can be slit open so easily like a bull pumped up for market, I thought, I only want life more, long to dance 'til my heart sweats, 'til my mind stops anticipating, 'til I understand the dead tree's part in the design. And having wept again, I realized that to be broken is no reason to see all things as broken. To fear death is not a calling.

Within weeks I had my first chemo treatment, which was horrific, vomiting blood every 20 minutes for 24 hours, my missing rib lancing me with every heave. For the next 3 weeks I vowed I would not continue, would never open my arm to that needle again. But in the dark center of my pain, an unwavering voice said, Poor, challenged man: the *treatment* is the miracle. And so, with more terror than I have ever known, I said yes and opened my arms to measured poisons. Finally, after 4 months of treatment, I sat in our wellness group where truth could relax its way out of hiding, and there I was asked to draw my cancer and my treatment, and suddenly I knew that the cancer was gone. Now the treatment was killing me, and the miracle appeared as the silent certainty with which I took my good doctor's hand and said, No, it's over. I won't do this anymore.

What a revelation—who would have guessed—that each situation demands a different aspect of miracle: visualizations, yes, craneotomy, no; visualizations, no, thoracic surgery, yes; chemo-cleansing, if I must, chemo-poison, no. And underneath it all, willful, constant prayer, an unrehearsed dialogue with God, as Martin Buber puts it. Still, even years later, we are never exempt from the fear and fragility. In truth, with the close of each day, I feel the vastness of night and know I still have love to fill it. But when the sun disappears, I am forced to accept that I can snuff in a gust, though I stay devoted to the art of flicker.

It is a constant challenge to find the current of life and to trust it, to behold the depth of what is until a relaxation of intent and anxiety allows us to find the spaces in our individuality that we then know as spirit. Only through the passageways of spirit can we be lifted when we are heavy and rinsed of the exaggerations of our fear.

---

*The Portable Blake, edited by Alfred Kazin. NY: Viking, 1946, p. 250.

Still, it is next to impossible to do this alone. We need the loving truth of others to be well. Inevitably, when one is *thrust* into life, into crisis, into transformation—without notice or instruction—some come with us and are forever changed while others watch as we are forced out to sea. It is the power of love that enables those who come along, and in truth, a language of experience is unearthed that cannot be translated to those who stay behind.

I learned this in an instant, 2 days after my rib surgery. You see, it was time. The tube had to come out. It had drained my lung of blood for days, through a slit in my side. The doctor was waiting and I looked to Paul at the foot of my bed. Without a word, he knew. All the talk of life was now in the steps between us. He made his way past the curtain. Our arms locked and he crossed over, no longer watching. He was *part* of the trauma and everything—the bedrail, the tube, my face, his face, the curve of blanket rubbing the tube, the doctor pulling the tube's length as I held onto Paul—everything pulsed. And I've since learned that if you want to create anything—peace of mind, a child, a painting of running water, a simple tier of lilies—you must cross over and hold. You must sweep past the curtain, no matter how clear. You must drop all reservations like magazines in waiting rooms. You must swallow your heart, leap across, and join.

This is one instance of many, and they all lead to one inescapable fact: sharing pain is the only way to stay alive. For the net of love helps absorb and distribute the struggle. It's taught me that if we share pain, which is a lot to ask, there is no room for pity. For the sharing of the struggle requires an investment, a real life-changing investment by those who care, an involvement that will instigate their own tandem suffering.

We are well today, because those who love us got involved, deeply involved, daily involved. And by being so healed, we are forever wed to their pain. We are forever open to their struggles. By being so loved, we can never shut our lives completely again. If they fall, we will live lower. If they rise, we will take on their dizziness. We will live like pools of water, each clearly individual but all sharing and exchanging the same slippage and rush of tides. Now I understand. This is the basis of human family: the sharing of pain, the investment of love by which we make a difference and are changed, again and again.

We are well because people didn't watch our suffering, but entered us and then felt love-sufferings of their own. At times, this hurt them too much, which, in turn, forced us to nurture them, until, in bare, essential ways on certain days, we weren't sure who was ill and who was well—a solution that saved us all.

During my odyssey with cancer, I learned a great many things. One of the most crucial was the almost simultaneous need to inhabit myself while staying connected with others. With each test and office visit and surgery and treatment, I had to prepare, as best I could, for things that no one could anticipate. But nonetheless, I had to center myself and connect with that flow of universe that fills me with a strength and perspective beyond my tiny self. In order to do this, I need to be alone. I need to enter my solitude, which once entered, becomes a threshold to everything that is elemental, eternal and divine. My wife and all my loved ones grew to expect my gathering inward, especially before each medical procedure. But once centered, once in the universal flow, I had to connect with my loved ones in order to endure the experience.

Now that I am well, the ways in which we survived alone together have stayed with me, and the more I have thought about them, the more they represent a basic and unavoidable paradox about living, which is this: Though each of us must go through our suffering alone, no one can make it alone. Though no one can save us from our own feelings, not one of us can carry those feelings in the world without the support of others.

I remember wheeling Anne to her surgery, her stretcher wobbling down the sanitized hall, her groggy eyes looking back at me, our hands entwined. I wheeled her as far as they would let me and then, quite suddenly, though I knew it was coming, the glass doors of the operating room stopped me and she was wheeled on. I stood there, pressed against the glass, watching her grow smaller and smaller.

I realized then that whether it be our search for purpose, our struggle with confusion, our working through grief, or the violent evolution of our identity, no one can go beyond the glass door with you. Each of us must do that work alone. Each of us must ask our questions and feel our pain and be surprised by wonder in the very personal terrain that exists beyond that glass door. The best we can do in loving others is wheel each other as far as possible and be there when our loved ones return. But the work that changes our very lives, the work that yields inner transformation, the work that allows us to be reborn within the same skin must always be done alone. This is the work of solitude, and the attending to and from the glass door is the work of compassion.

Yet how do we access the flow and miracle of the whole? How can we, when broken, open ourselves to all that is not broken? It all begins with faith—faith in everything larger than the singular self. And it helps to remember that faith is inextricably linked to care.

As the theologian Paul Tillich contends, "Faith is the state of being ultimately concerned, an act of the total personality. It is the most centered act of the human mind."* So faith is no more than the willingness and bravery to be ultimately concerned, fueling that concern with everything that matters. The mystery is that taking the risk to be so ultimately concerned *in itself* makes us more whole, and what is compassion but being ultimately concerned about something other than ourselves.

In actuality, miracle is the process of ultimate concern, and one aspect of miracle is what happens when love makes us cross over into the sharing of each other's pain. Mysteriously and powerfully, when I look deeply enough into you, I find me, and when you dare to hear my fear in the recess of your heart, you recognize it as your secret, which you thought no one else knew. And that unexpected wholeness that is more than each of us, but common to all—that moment of unity—is the atom of God.

This all became clear to me as I was sitting tired, nervous, and afraid in a waiting room at Columbia Presbyterian Hospital in New York City, staring straight into this old Hispanic woman's eyes, she into mine. In our desperate stare I accepted that we all see the same wonder, all feel the same agony, though we all speak in a different voice.

Suddenly, I knew that each being born, inconceivable as it seems, is another Adam or Eve, each of us unique and common. Suddenly I understood that the most essential things I perceive and feel, we all feel. And now, in truth, I believe this acceptance is helping me stay alive.

I will never forget that burdened majestic Hispanic grandmother fighting her tumor as she looked at me across the waiting room without a word on that sweltering day, the way an old Egyptian slave at one oar must have looked at his younger counterpart three oars down: no pretense, no manners, no needed phrases, but simply a tired soul that would not look away, saying, Though this body is chained, these eyes are your eyes and they are forever free.

In that moment, we became the truth we were painfully entering, the way a diver against his will becomes the deep. In the wash of silence that emptied our hearts, we were the still point of eternity. In that moment of ultimate concern, across the stained and sterilized corridors, at the core, we were healed because, without knowing each other's name, our spirits were one.

■

Dynamics of Faith, Paul Tillich. NY: Harper and Brothers, 1957, p. 4.

I am often asked how I account for the tumor vanishing from my head. I can only answer from *inside the miracle*. I can only begin by retelling what the ancient Chinese philosopher Chuang Tzu believed when he said, "Great knowledge sees all in one. Small knowledge breaks down into the many."* I can only whisper that like the deepest wind, it will move us all and remain unseen. I know that just as everyone else wanted to blame this illness on their partial understanding of disease: it's in your bones, in your food, in the synthetics of your home, the vinyl of your Pontiac, in the emptiness of your life, it's in your protein, in your spinal fluid, in your lack of vitamins, it's in your sexuality, in your stress, in your family, your century, your water, your air.

Just so. And I know that everyone will claim its disappearance for their partial understanding of wellness: it was Jesus, it was Moses, it was our collective prayers, it was the strength of your mind, it was your visualization, your writing, your goodness returning to you, it was the technology of the day, the medicine of the day, the expertise of your doctors, your change in diet, your change in outlook, your ability to endure, your ability to submit, your ability to take charge, your capacity to accept, it was our love for you, it was your love of life.

Just so. It has been our lot since the conception of consciousness to praise what we are and blame what we are not. Yet I have been blessed to have a Catholic priest lay his brooding hands on my Jewish head. I have had a woman I've never met lead a Sufi meditation weekly on my behalf. I have had an artist paint his version of Michelangelo to give me strength. And a poet made a bookmark of sweet grass meant to heal. And I have had deep friends pull crystals from the earth and wash them for me to carry as protection. And yet another has given us a petal from the Philippines that appeared in a miracle in 1948. And old friends in New Hampshire have designed a cancer-free diet that they are assuming with us. And my brother is insisting that I exercise and consume vast quantities of vitamin C. And a kind woman who has loved us from afar enrolled us both in the daily prayers of yet another religious order in Massachusetts. And a sweet friend who does not believe in God sits with me in silence when I have nothing left to say. And still another dear soul is praying to her dead mother and to Thomas Merton that we be healed. And I even talk to Grandma sometimes or visualize in her golden chairs.

Just so. I am blessed that all these efforts carry me. For each is indispensable. Just so. I need Catholic, Jew, Mystic, Sweet Grass, Sufi, Herbs, Crystal, Dead Mother, Dead Grandmother, Dead Monk, and Golden Chairs to heal.

I know only that everything has helped and I am not great enough or wise enough to break down into percentages how much vitamin, how much medicine, how much prayer, how much God, how much Jesus, and how much mental fight. I know only that those who suffer partial belief are only partially healed.

I know only that I have been loved into wholeness, beyond my stubborn flaws. I know only that pain has pried me open to the freedom of spirit that forms the spokes of the world. I know only that unconditional love brought eternity to my lip. I know only that alone we each spread like a wing and that together we can fly.

It is no secret that cancer in its acuteness pierced me into open living, and I've been working ever since to sanctify that open port without crisis as its trigger. But can this be done without crisis pushing us off the ledge? That's the question now, years from the leap: how to keep leaping from a desire to be real so as not to be shoved by an ever-lurking crisis.

---

*The Basic Writings of Chuang Tzu, translated by Burton Watson. NY: Columbia University Press, 1964.

In essence, when broken, survival is the standing watch. But once broken into wholeness, living is blessing every crack as an opening, treasuring the song that whistles through as God, praying the break to let him in won't end it all.

And I for one confess: I started after power, not over others but like a raw element, like wind bending maples, but now I want the sweetness of a delicate hour, the light burning through an abandoned web. How do I give you where I've been. How do I open my palms and say, See how pain has simplified the air, see how struggle has boiled down to joy. They say that birds dream in the nest and whatever they see makes them wake and sing. How late must it be for me to whisper that our nest is our suffering. How quiet for me to offer that living is in the vastness that experience opens. How utterly rearranged must we be to realize that loving is the courage to hold each other as we break and worship what unfolds.

LONG-TERM CARE

When I asked if it hurt
he waited a long time,
then pointed with his eyes
to some scene he alone could see:
"Note how the hawk hooks
the thinnest branch."

I knew better than to prod him.
Several minutes later, he
surfaced again: "It waits
for something real to move."

He closed his eyes:
"The heart is a big red blind
hawk. It hooks the thinnest bone."

He was suddenly in pain.
I took his hand. The nurse came.
He squeezed me hard, then
let go: "There, the hawk has fed.
I can rest."

I watched him from my chair
in the dark. When he slept,
the hawk was in flight.

THE MUSIC BENEATH THE MUSIC

I have tried so hard to please
that I never realized
no one is watching.

I imagined like everyone at school
that our parents were sitting
just out of view like those
quiet doctors behind clean mirrors.

I even felt the future
gather like an audience,
ready to marvel at how much
we had done with so little.

But when I woke bleeding after surgery
with all those mothlike angels
breathing against me, I couldn't
talk and the audience was gone.

I cried way inside and the sobs
were no more than the water
of a deshelled spirit
breaking ground.

Years have passed and I wait
long hours in the sun to see the birch
fall of its own weight into the lake
and it seems to punctuate God's mime.

Nothing sad about it.

And sometimes, at night,
when the dog is asleep
and the owl is beginning to stare
into what no one ever sees,
I stand on the deck and feel
the black spill off the stars,
feel it coat the earth, the trees,
the minds of children half alseep,
feel the stlllness evaporate
like notions of fame
into light.

CRITICAL-THINKING ACTIVITIES

1. Describe Mark Nepo's initial experience of fear when he learned that he had cancer. Discuss the power of fear psychologically and spiritually.

2. In a dream the author asked the Chinese poet Tu Fu, "How do I block the fear?" Tu Fu answers his question with another: "How does a tree block the wind?" How, exactly, did this dream help the author to endure and recover from fear?

3. How is the knowledge imparted by Tu Fu useful to you in your personal and professional life?

4. How might the isolation and power of fear inhibit the relationship between practitioner and patient?

5. The author explores different types of suffering in this narrative. What are they and how are they intertwined?

6. Do you find that patients ask in anguish, "Why is there all of this suffering?" Compare how they voice this with the author's narrative.

7. Do you agree with the author that while suffering threatens life, it can also enrich it? Discuss your response in detail.

8. Does the notion of *valuing suffering* surprise you? Explain.

9. Discuss in detail the physiological effects of prayer, visualization, and meditation, using current scientific literature.

10. Is there a dual nature in all of us? How do you understand this paradox or mystery? How can we be, according to the author, both weak and strong? Afraid and brave? Resilient and stalled? Confused and clear? Could we be all of these things at the same time? How would this knowledge affect the way in which you approach patients?

11. How is the writer's experience of suffering transformed into hope and distilled in his poems?

Rebecca Sachs Norris

Rebecca Sachs Norris is currently a PhD candidate in mythology and comparative religion at Boston University. She is married and has two children. Her other areas of interest include music, weaving, and lace making. Before entering graduate school, she had a small gourmet baking business. Before starting a family she was a computer programmer and systems analyst.

Here Norris shares a gift of infinite value from her dying friend: the growing understanding of the potential of illness as a force of life and a part of life.

CHAPTER 15

For Gabe and Ari

by Rebecca Sachs Norris

*T*he experiences of many of the women I have met who are about the same age as I am, and who early in life experienced the loss of someone close, have been very similar. A number of these women I met through the death of a mutual friend. That event opened the possibility of a different experience of death, a different relation to it for family and friends.

My mother died 5 days after my 16th birthday, after a long struggle with breast cancer. She left behind my father and five children ranging in age from 8 to 22. Her illness had initially been kept secret from my younger siblings and myself; I understand now that this was common practice in those days. When I was about 10 years old I found out from a friend (whom I did not believe) that my mother had cancer. Our family's relationship to her illness was one of pain and fear, a closing.

My friend J's illness (metastasized inflammatory breast cancer), with all its highs and lows, took place unhidden in the very center of her family. A bed was set up in the living room when she became too ill from disease and treatment to use the second floor. This way, she was always part of the family activity, able to be present for her two children and husband. Even when painful, or frightening, her illness and the possibility of her death were a part of her life, a part of family life, and a part of the natural course of the universe.

J understood her illness as intimately linked with her spiritual growth. I do not say this lightly, nor do I mean it in any New Age mumbo-jumbo sense. Her struggle in her relationship with her suffering was the ultimate struggle of spirit and body, of the meaning of life and death. We spoke about it once as the hero's journey, the subject of myth as well as religion, the ultimate challenge. It was as though she had been abruptly removed from the normal course of life and dropped into the middle of a maelstrom— the heroine who falls down the well into another world, Alice in Wonderland, where one can never quite figure out the sense of the new world or catch up to it. Perhaps I should say, rather, that the sense of this new world is of a completely different order from that of the old world.

Every decision in this new world can be, and often is, a life-and-death decision. There are more choices and more information than ever before, and if one treatment doesn't work, then the next decision must be made, so that the excruciating difficulty of these decisions occurs repeatedly. I remember how relieved J was whenever some decision, *any* decision, had been made.

During the course of her illness she kept a journal and started working with painting. These were both part of her journey of self-discovery. Her spiritual growth and deepening can be felt in her artwork as a palpable force.

She died at home, with her family and friends around her. Her children were not kept away, but included. She faced her death with courage and with faith; one can truly say that she died well. Until now I could not have conceived that such an attitude toward death was possible; it is certainly not a common idea. Generally, when the question of living wills or sudden death arises, the common consensus is that no suffering is good suffering and one should go as quickly as possible. How different to have witnessed J's inner growth and unfolding!

When I arrived at her home shortly after she died, her body was on the bed in the living room, and there was a presence in the room that can only be described by that word—presence. Throughout the day she had a smile on her face.

Helping to take care of her body and dress her (since those close to her would be coming by during the day) felt like something we could do for her, out of love and respect. It was not awful to touch her body (remember, I am not in a medical profession and had never touched a dead body before). It was simply a body with the life separated from it. This, in part, is what that feeling of presence was, the sensing of life, separated from the body. At the same time it was more than that, for it was not so much a personal feeling, that J's spirit or life force was still in the room with us, but rather a deeper or higher sense of presence, of life force greater than the individual.

After the funeral many of her friends and family returned to her house. A few hours later a number of us came together to share stories and experiences of J's life. There was laughter as well as tears, joy in her living as well as sadness in her dying. Her children were there as well, hearing how their mother was loved and missed, not in a somber, solemn tone, but with funny stories, poetry, whatever a person had to offer. What they also saw was the sharing of life, the adults facing the cycle of life together, without turning away or denying any part of it.

In her dying J gave us each a gift of infinite value. Even before her death I knew that my growing understanding of the potential of illness as a force of life and a part of life had altered something deep in me. When I was faced with a breast biopsy (I never told J about it) while she was in the midst of intensive chemotherapy and radiation treatments, I knew that it was possible to face either outcome as my *life*, as an opening rather than a closing. I was no longer bound by my experience of my mother's illness. Suffering may be an opportunity to face a deeper part of ourselves, a part we all must face sooner or later since we are all mortal. And that suffering may be necessary for our transformation, to help us realize, in the sense of "making real," a more profound, inner experience of life. In this we may be assisting the interpenetration of higher and lower, truly bringing the sacred into our lives.

At the gathering following J's funeral I read the following excerpt from a letter that Pierre Teilhard de Chardin wrote to his sister, who had long been ill:

> O Marguerite, my sister, while I, given soul and body to the positive forces of the universe, was wandering over continents and oceans, my whole being passionately taken up in watching the intensification of the world's tints and shadows, you were lying motionless, stretched out on your bed of sickness, silently, deep within yourself, transforming into light the world's most grievous shadows. In the eyes of the Creator, which of us, tell me, which of us will have had the better part?

CRITICAL-THINKING ACTIVITIES

1. Does the knowledge of the way that J faced her suffering and death affect your view of the value of suffering? How is this so?

2. Examine the implications of viewing J's illness as linked to her spiritual growth. How would this affect her struggle in "her relationship to her suffering"?

3. What did the author experience as she witnessed this woman's courage and faith?

4. Could you comment on the presence in J's room throughout the day of her death? Have you ever experienced such a presence when caring for the dead?

5. What gift of infinite value did the author's dying friend give her family and friends? How does this influence your approach to facing the death of someone close to you?

6. Discuss the importance of the gathering of family and friends to share stories and the experience of J's life. What are the many positive and long-term effects of this?

Linda Q. Trott

Linda Q. Trott is a clinical nurse specialist with a BS in nursing from
Boston University School of Nursing and an MS in psychiatric and mental
health nursing from the University of Massachusetts School of Nursing at
Amherst. She is the director of clinical services and associate area director
for a health-care company responsible for managing the mental health and
substance abuse treatment for 450,000 individuals. She has authored
articles about managed mental health care and care in the home. She has
presented her research on the psychiatrically ill treated at home at the
National Managed Health Care Congress in Washington, DC.

Linda Trott shares excerpts from the personal journal she kept while
caring for her dying friend, Jean. The subtle but sure tracings of the facets
of compassion visible in the interchanges between these two women offer
unique insights into its process and workings.

CHAPTER 16

Journey with a Friend

by Linda Q. Trott

November 1994: It has been 14 months since Jean died, and I am now ready to share our experience. The power of the experience of being with a friend and colleague through the final days of her life cannot be captured in print. But I hope that by sharing the experience, I might be able to help someone else faced with the death of a friend, loved one, or patient accept the natural and inevitable final chapter of that person's life without fear or avoidance, and to be a part of it. So often, people would comment on how wonderful it was that I cared for and was with my friend through her dying and give me undue praise and acknowledgement. But it is I who feel humbled to have been allowed by my friend to share in such an intimate and personal experience, which would ultimately change my life forever, and it is I who am grateful for what she gave me. If I can convey that message of the wonderment of giving of oneself to be with another during her death experience, then I feel that I will have given something back in return for all that I have received.

I allowed myself the experience. I trusted through the panic, and I risked the pain because I was fortunate to be coached by my friend as she was dying; she mentored me along, guiding me on how to help her through her death experience, and so I want also to share what she taught me.

She became the master, and I became her student, and we learned from each other as we progressed through the experience. We talked about writing of our experience together in her daily journey as she battled to survive her cancer, and she asked that I finish the book if anything ever happened to her, and I promised that I would.

In 1988, I casually went for a job interview at a health insurance company, at the time called a health maintenance organization (HMO) or managed-care company, for a position as a mental health nurse case manager. I was interviewed by several members from management; my final encounter was with Jean, who was commissioned to interview me as a prospective colleague. We immediately had a common bond: we had both graduated from Boston University School of Nursing in the late 1960s and had both entered the field of mental health nursing. I was struck by her warmth, her professionalism, and her intelligence. Regal, majestic, dignified, engaging, and yet intimidating with her self-confidence and eloquent manner of communicating, she intrigued me. I was struck as well by her gentleness and could feel her support of me in the middle of a tedious series of interviews for the position.

Within a few weeks, I joined the staff of nurse case managers, all with our own clinical specialities; Jean and I became the two mental health case managers. Jean managed all the HMO members in need of alcohol or substance abuse treatment, and I managed all the members in need of psychiatric services. As members frequently need both treatments, Jean and I developed a very close working relationship, consulting with one another and covering each other's cases as needed. So began our relationship as professionals and colleagues in the health insurance world of the late 1980s. Surely our paths had crossed some 20 years earlier in nursing school in Boston, but neither of us were aware of that, or of what lay ahead. What was significant was that we had experienced the same training with the same professors, textbooks, and model of nursing, and we felt total confidence in each other's practice style, expertise, and philosophy of care. This was significant as we worked closely as colleagues developing a managed mental health care program for the HMO, but it would become even more significant when I transitioned from colleague to nurse and caregiver.

I was initially quite taken with Jean—graduate of the prestigious Boston University School of Nursing, daughter of a minister who had once been chaplain at Princeton University. I enjoyed watching her, listening to her talk on the phone to acutely ill alcoholics and substance abusers in need of treatment, and observing her creativity in planning care. I actually looked forward to going in to work on Monday mornings just to be able to learn from her. She had been doing case management for 2 years when I entered this subspeciality, and she became my mentor and teacher. Our relationship was strictly professional, as she did not mix social life with work; in fact, the other nurses found her rather reserved and unsociable. They would comment on not understanding why she would often work through lunch hours, or not join the group for social events after work or around the coffee machine; they saw her as much too serious. But I was mystified by her; How could she be so consistently dedicated to and focused on her work, so pure and good? She never vacillated. It was beyond my comprehension, for I had not experienced anyone like this before; she truly loved her work and gave every individual she spoke to her undivided attention and the best plan of care she could. She never complained about her heavy workload or about any of the difficult cases, which could be very tedious at times and wear anyone else's patience a bit thin—but not Jean. Colleagues would express annoyance at her "perfection," and though I could understand their not understanding her, I would be irritatied with the comments and would try to defend her. At the same time, I would talk to Jean about loosening up a little, about the importance of being more socially involved with her colleagues, about the importance of taking lunch breaks, because I genuinely liked her, in addition to admiring her competence and dedication, and wanted her to be a part of the group.

Within a few months of my joining the company, Jean confided in me that she was a cancer survivor; 5 years earlier she had been diagnosed with non-Hodgkin's lymphoma and had been treated with chemotherapy and radiation. I was a bit frightened to hear of her diagnosis and also intrigued to hear about her successful treatment. And because she had been symptom-free for 5 years, I was confident that she was cured and would live a full life like anyone else who had no history of cancer. I did not give it much more thought, but felt touched that she could share such personal information with me, knowing how private she kept her personal life. I would sometimes look at her and think about her situation as a cancer survivor, but would assure myself that the cancer was not likely to recur because of the magic 5 years without symptoms.

Six months into my employment, Jean complained of a sore throat that would not go away. She was diagnosed with a recurrence of the lymphoma at a new primary site. At work she told me first and asked me to help inform our peers in a group setting, so we could tell everyone at once. We did. I was angry and scared, and decided to deny the seriousness of this second episode. I felt she could conquer this again as she had done once before. I made myself available to her whenever she needed to talk, whether at work, after work, or by phone at home. I was committed to supporting her through this crisis.

She was, as always, amazing. She continued to work around the chemotherapy and radiation treatments on a part-time basis. Though relatively new at my position, I covered all the mental health and substance abuse cases so her responsibilities would be met and there would be no problem with management and job security, no matter how much time she needed for treatments or recuperation. No matter how tired or how weakened she became from the treatments, she was always available for consultation by phone and remained concerned about her clients, asking for updates on their progress in treatment. As her own treatment progressed, she became very tired, thin, and physically ill, but, true to form, she continued to come in to work, even if just for a couple of hours a week. Sometimes, on the weekend, she would have her companion drive her in to get some work, so she could prepare reports at home to meet a deadline. She lost all her hair and transitioned to a wig without missing a beat. Many people outside the department had no idea what this galant woman was going through. She continued to care for her clients. She worried when they didn't comply with treatment or talked about suicide. I would feel angry that she was struggling for life while they talked to her about wanting to die, but she never faltered in her professionalism and handled her cases with unending care, even when she was ill herself from the side effects of the treatment.

I was unnerved when I first saw her cry as she spoke of her fear. She was always a pillar of strength, and it made me feel so helpless to help her, as she continued to help others. But I encouraged her to talk and told her she would never go through this alone; I wanted nothing more than to support her while she returned to wellness. I never once thought that she might not survive. Jean felt my support, as she began to address me in her journal, writing, "Dear Journal/Linda." I felt honored that she would share something so intimate with me, and yet at the same time did not want to deal with the emotions of anguish and fear that she was expressing. So I would read the journal as she gave it to me, and then I would put it away in an unmarked manilla envelope, which I would hide out of sight on the bottom shelf of a bookcase. Even now, I can remember how I felt when she gave me her writings: I wanted to read them and be supportive but her emotional pain and fear were too much to bear, so by quickly putting the manuscripts away, I could deny that her situation was so bad. I actually would skim the journal, thinking that this would be easier than reading it closely. I would feel guilty, but I was uncertain how I could help her and felt unable to change her situation. And I was certain she would survive, so we did not have to feel so sad. She was a survivor.

And survive she did. For another 5 years, we worked together; I became her supervisor when our department expanded and restructured, but we remained equal colleagues and professionals. She was strong and consistent and a wonderful mental health nurse. As a two-time cancer survivor, she became more vocal about her illness and a major support to people in similar situations. She became as involved with cancer cases as with her substance abuse cases, and received a state award for her cancer support group work. Sometimes, I felt that I did not want to hear about cancer anymore. It was over and I wanted to move on.

Jean continued to be a support to everyone around her, to be perfect in the way she did her work, and to be forever grateful for every day and every friend. She never spoke harshly or negatively about anyone, and saw the good in everything; she focused on strengths and the positive to a point where some felt she was phoney, that no one could be so nice and "perfect" all the time. But as I observed her, I came to realize that she was very much for real; I know now that she had faced the prospect of imminent death twice, and that every day truly was a gift for her. She was for real.

I also saw her as indestructable. So when she wanted to talk about cancer or how precious every moment of life was, I did not give her the full attention I came to realize much later she deserved. It may have been my denial that she might not be indestructable. She would send me the most beautifully written notes and cards telling me how important our professional relationship and friendship were to her. She would make me feel that I had done so much for her, when in fact, I had done very little. And I would feel guilty that I was not the good person she thought I was, but rather someone who kept just enough detached to deny that she could ever fall out of remission.

For 5 years, we worked very closely together every day. We would talk about personal matters, especially as related to our adolescent children. On occasion, we would go to lunch; Jean became much more interested in our spending time together in later years, but I had become more aloof and took her being there so consistently and supportively for granted, and would not be as available as I had been initially.

Around Thanksgiving, 1992, Jean began to complain that her stomach bothered her. She saw her doctor, but nothing abnormal was found. Jean commented on how a cancer survivor gets a minor ailment like the flu or a stomach upset, and everyone immediately suspects the worst. She was relieved that her problem was just a routine ailment unrelated to cancer. I felt a little suspicious, but kept my thoughts to myself. Shortly thereafter, she complained about a pain in her groin, following a few days of strenous walking for exercise. A day later, she noticed a lump in the area and suspected a pulled muscle. She nursed the pain herself for a few days with no relief. I was scared and suggested maybe she should see her doctor. After a multitude of tests, she called me at home to tell me that she had a new malignancy. This time she cried and cried. She sounded so defeated, and I felt that gnawing ache in the gut I had never thought I would feel about Jean's condition. She started chemotherapy right after the holidays—whopping doses of chemotherapy for 5 days on an inpatient basis every 4 weeks for a few months and then a bone marrow transplant. She went on medical leave, and I kept her position open for her eventual return to work while the rest of the staff and I covered her case load. We managed to keep the position open for 8 months.

From January to June 1993, I was in continuous contact with Jean by phone. Whenever she was hospitalized, I would be there to see her. Initially, she was very upbeat and optimistic, but as treatments progressed, she became very weak and tired. Sometimes, I would just sit outside her hospital door on my way home from work or on a lunch hour without even telling her I was there, as I knew that she would feel she would have to be cordial and sociable no matter how bad she felt. I never gave up hope that she would make it to transplant, but something about this time was different. The gnawing in my gut never went away.

She was a very private person. I had been to her home only once, when she invited me to dinner to celebrate my master's degree. I did not feel comfortable going by her home without an invitation. Ours was a formal friendship. Jean was a very private person and kept her personal life very separate from work. I was her colleague and her boss. But in late July 1993, I asked if I could stop by to see her at her home.

When I arrived, Roger, Jean's companion for the past 17 years, went out to get Chinese food for dinner. Jean and I had time to catch up on all that she was currently going through—the numerous phone calls from caring and well-meaning friends and family, her increasing fatigue, her inability to take walks around the neighborhood that had always provided her so much pleasure, her hope for a bone marrow transplant, her reality that it might not happen, her concern for Roger and her two grown children, Kristin, 21, and Daren, 23. When Roger returned, we had a lovely dinner at the elegantly set dining room table. Later we sat outside on the back deck. The evening was pleasantly warm, so peaceful and enjoyable, and I was relieved to see my friend in the comfort of her home after so many weeks instead of the oncology unit in the hospital, the only place I had seen her for the past 6 months. When it was time to go home, Jean walked me to my car, and as I was about to back out of the driveway, she said, "Love you." I replied so naturally, "I love you, too, Jean." Something was very different. After I returned home, I wrote the following letter.

FRIDAY

JULY 30, 1993

Dear Jean,

I so enjoyed my evening with you, Roger, and Ippin [their black Labrador dog]. I could barely wait to see you, and once there, I felt so happy and relieved to see you all.

On my drive home [25 miles], my mind was flooded with thoughts so that I was transported beyond the trip home and now find myself sitting on my sofa with little recollection of the actual maneuver of driving home. I expect it was like a deep meditation. It happens, for example, sometimes when I run; I know you can relate to this experience.

Anyway, among my thoughts was the recollection of your "journaling" me the last time you were ill and how close that made me feel to you and your experience. . . . And how now I want to journal you about my experience in relation to you this time. You say you have been doing a bit of reading; for a moment, put down your books, and read this.

In the comfort of your home with you and Roger, I felt time stand still—a wonderful rare experience. Being able to talk without interruption and to share thoughts and each other's presence was so refreshing. To be able to talk about your plans for death, your plans for life was so natural and free. It struck me at how alive you are—hear me—not at how well you look and act and all that superficial stuff, but how truly alive you are—more so than anyone else I know. It is enviable the depth of your living. So when I am with you, I celebrate life and feel alive with you. And I feel we all can do the same with death, the final stage of this life; experience what is with open honesty. I am in awe of your capacity for life, and how alive you "enable" me to feel. I can cut through the falseness and feel the depth of my emotion without condition with you. That's being alive. Thank you.

It did my heart good to see you eat and enjoy your Chinese food, as I know how queasy you have been the past few weeks. You are taking such good care of yourself with your elastic stockings, leg elevated, good temperature control, and everything just the way it should be done; Roger takes good care of you too. Your love for each other is so beautifully obvious; you are fortunate.

Jean, I can't tell you how important it was for me to hear about your plans for what will happen if you live or if you die. I am pleased and relieved to have your sister's name and phone number; as you would say, "Thank you for sharing."

I think a lot lately about life, relationships; about my being "alone" at work without you, which lends me even more time for introspection. I wonder why I miss you so much, and why we didn't spend more "quality time" together like at lunch or maybe after work, etc. Part of the reason was my preoccupation with family matters, which was a reality. But I have come up with other ideas. I felt a closeness to you that I never felt a need to talk about or to nurture—it just was—and I also took your "being there" for granted. Your consistency, your loyalty lets people like me flounder about and float with the tide, knowing the security of the mooring is and will be there for stabilizing when the seas get rough. I regret that selfishness, and I am sorry; but I have learned. I am learning not to take anything for granted, and ah-h-h-h that I too can be a securing and stabilizing force; and I want to be there for you, as you have been there so often for so many others, including me. When you return to work, we will lunch regularly, at least.

You know what else I miss, Jean—at work—is your professionalism, your elegance, and your consistent dedication and honesty. They just don't put out nurses like you anymore! I try to emulate your example, but I just don't quite make it. Keep teaching us.

Enough for one sitting. Let me say, I thoroughly enjoyed our dinner, our talk, our visit, and just being with you and Roger.

I do not speak of love often, I don't even sign cards and letters with "love" routinely. I am reserved and selective, and sincere, as are you. So our parting words expressing a loving bond between us meant a lot to me. I respect you. I respect our special relationship.

Friends forever

Love,

Linda

And so began my journal of our final 3 months together. From the night I wrote this letter, I continued to write in a notebook raw material about our experience together. I would feel compelled to write, especially when I felt deeply emotional, and knew not where to turn or how to express all that I was feeling in such depth. I shared what I wrote with no one; the act of writing was a very private matter, and it provided a comfort I never dreamed possible. I would carry the journal around with me, and other than being with Jean, I would want to be with my journal. It helped to stabilize me and provide some clarity about all that was happening so quickly. I never planned to share the journal with anyone but maybe Jean one day, and never went back to reread what I had written until now, 14 months after her death.

She was a remarkable woman. She lived a remarkable life. She died a remarkable death. And yet in reality, quite simply, she is no different from anyone else; nor is her experience: we all live, we all die. Our journeys vary, and whom we invite to take along, or whom we agree to go along with, varies; but we all experience life and life's end. Jean invited me on her journey and I wanted to go, and she gave me a most precious gift. In return, I want to share the experience of this "journey with a friend," so that others might understand and embrace the beauty and honor of the invitation.

The Journal

AUGUST 7, 1993

It's a still night. I visited with Jean and Roger this Saturday afternoon into the evening, having been in their company last Friday, July 30. Roger prepared a wonderful chicken dinner with fresh vegetables and corn on the cob. Roger has a corn butterer that is truly unique, and it gave us something superficial to talk about as we began our evening together.

As dinner progressed, we talked about how Jean and Roger met and fell in love over 17 years ago. They both took pleasure in describing the events leading to their finally moving in together. Then Jean turned the conversation to his and her going to see a counselor to talk about grief and pain, to put it simply. She tried to make him talk about what was worrying him. He cried at the dinner table as he talked about not being able to make her better, his feeling of loss of control. She expresses worry about him, his loss of weight, his sadness, his not talking to anyone about this. He contradicts her by saying he talks to James, Jean's beloved brother in New York, and he assures her he's talking now. Following Jean's cue for my assistance, I encourage him to go with Jean to see a professional. He agrees to go with her. We then proceed to indulge in a chocolate cream pie, which I had brought, but I, of all three, have the hardest time eating. I too feel helpless, and want so desperately to be able to comfort and make things better. I understand what Roger is feeling.

Jean tells me it was hard for James to see her when he visited this past week, for she is debilitated now and looks so different from when he last saw her 3 months ago at a family wedding. He is doing well; she helped him through a very difficult time when he had some emotional problems a few months before she became ill this last time. He had been her priority; even at work she would talk with him on the phone—the only time she ever tended to a personal matter at work—only for James. Even when she was ill 5 years ago, through all Roger's medical problems over the years, with the turmoil of her kids' adolescence—she never abused work time to deal with personal matters. She cries, as she recalls. I agree; there are times when your priority is cut-and-dried, without question, and I remind her of how important she was to James at that time in his life. Erika, my daughter, phones to tell me she will be out for the evening; Kristin, Jean's daughter, phones to check on her more. I ask to speak to Kristin and playfully scold her for not coming by to see me; she has a party to go to. She thanks me for being with her mom and tells me her mom sounds so much better when I am there. I tell her we (she and I) must get together. She agrees. Jean's sister-in-law calls; I go outside onto the back deck with Roger, to afford Jean privacy as she talks with her sister-in-law.

I confide in Roger how I cry every day on the way to and from work, and how I sometimes want to call him just to check in. He thanks me for coming by this night. He talks about what he will do, where he will live. I see he is preparing, clearly more than Jean is aware. I tell her later, for she is so worried about Roger and what he will do, and I feel it is important for her to know that he is thinking about the future more than she knows. She says she is at peace and wants him to be as well. Earlier we talked about grief, and I remarked on grief being the price we pay for love. Roger tells me about his two previous marriages and some hard breaks he has endured through his life. He is kind and gentle, and I am pleased to be getting to know him.

I hear Jean crying inside while she is talking on the phone, and I feel so sorry she has to go through the story of her treatment regime with everyone, and the energy it takes from her. But she wants to keep everybody informed, to fulfill their need to know the details. She joins Roger and me on the deck and tries to enter casually into our conversation as if nothing is wrong, avoiding what she has just experienced inside. She is out of breath and I tell her to take a few deep breaths and place my hand on her shoulder. She looks at me with annoyance and continues to talk. I think to myself: "Oh, oh. Let her be." We move on to talk about music. Roger is musical and has a large repertoire of old songs and jingles; they reminisce about his singing to the children at night when they were little, a special song for each one after evening prayers. He sings the songs for me. I enjoyed it so, especially the expression on Jean's face as she remembers tenderly the nightly routine with her children so many years ago. It was a wonderful moment. The mosquitoes bite; we go inside.

Jean lies on the couch to raise her swollen right leg with the enlarged lymph nodes. We continue to talk. Roger says I am a comfort to them in their home. I say they are a comfort to me. Roger says I give so much. Me? I say he and Jean give to me. Roger goes outside. I ask Jean privately what I can do for her. She wants me to handle telling people when she dies; of course, I will. Martha, her sister, will tell the family. I will tell the people at work and Jean's multitude of friends. We talk of a plan to get a list together. I assure her I will handle it. I do not cry as we talk, but my insides tremble. She cries as she tells of so many who write her and starts naming them all, as if she does not want any of them left off the list. I say we will get the list together. She talks about being okay now, but questions what will happen when she needs care. I can't even imagine her getting to a point when she will need care; but I say I will be available, 24 hours a day, if need be. She cries and looks me in the eye, and says that that means a lot. Roger returns. I assure them both I am involved; I am invested. No one else understands this experience. Jean thanks me for being on the journey. I say, as I said 5 years ago, "You will never journey alone." She is tired, and the nights are hardest, as she has told me. I remind her that each night turns into a beautiful dawn. She needs rest; it is hard to leave. I try to lighten the conversation as I prepare to leave. I tell Roger he makes good coffee; he smiles. I pick up a little, putting cups in the sink; I am comfortable in their home. I go to the couch to hug Jean and tell her I love her. (A relationship changes so quickly when time is limited.) After a long embrace, I look into her eyes and she is crying hard. I put my hands on her shoulders, firmly look her in the eyes and tell her we will get through this. She talked earlier about when to put a halt to the needles and technology and medicines, and she and Roger agreed they would decide together. I am not ready yet to give up hope. We will take it one day at a time. I hug Roger. He follows me outside and says thank you again and again. I thank him. I am able to drive home without crying, unlike last week, when I cried all the way home. Writing this journal helps me to know where we have been and where we are going. She gives so much; she has given me more than I can express. I want to ease her struggle and be there for her.

AUGUST 12, 1993

It has only been 6 days since I last wrote. But so much has happened.

Last Sunday, August 8, I took my daughter Erika, a freshman at the University of Connecticut (UConn), back to school, coincidentally 5 miles from Jean and Roger's home. (I am beginning to think there is something to be said for fate—my daughter enrolls in a college 5 miles away from Jean's home and begins just as I start spending time at Jean's.) I called Jean. She invited me over, as I had hoped she would. She was lying on the couch, all in light blue, and looked so peaceful, but tired. We talked lightly, the three of us, and Roger offered me gourmet peanut butter pie, made by their neighbor. I had planned to stay only 10 minutes or so, but Jean said that the children would be home soon from an excursion with their father. Kristin and Daren, Jean's grown children, and Reid, Kristin's boyfriend, came in within 30 minutes of my arrival, very excited and energized from having been tubing down some large river in Connecticut; they were full of stories to share. Jean questioned them at length about their experience, and she came to life with her interest in their day. Roger talked about growing up in Lake Placid, and being on a bobsled team as a young man. They all reminisce about how Jean and Roger and the kids had planned to go to the Olympics there and how they had all gotten sick; they went on and on about fun times the family had shared together through the years. Daren sat on a dining room chair placed near Jean lying on the couch, but I could not help but notice a certain aloofness on his part. Jean places her hand on his knee. Kristin sits on the living room rug, and Reid collapses in an easy chair. There is plenty of family talk and liveliness. Jean had had Roger turn up the lights before the kids walked into the house to make the room bright and cheery, and it was indeed that. I get up to leave, as I recognize the need for their private family time, too. I hug Jean good-bye and tell her I love her, and she holds me tight. Roger comes over and he hugs me with gratitude. Then Jean tells Kristin to give me a hug, too, and Reid, and Daren. The boys are awkward and a bit uncomfortable, as was I, I suppose: we didn't even know each other.

Earlier Jean had told Kristin to show me her bedroom and the new curtains they had put up in her room. Jean is making connections, tying the knots for when she leaves us all behind in sorrow. She is such a remarkable woman. I never cease to marvel at her. I leave and feel good to have connected with Jean's beautiful family, and I daydream of my family joining in fun with her and hers one day. I also know she is very tired, and she feels bloated, like she is constipated, but knows she is not, like there is something growing inside her. She is uncomfortable and lies down to feel less pressure in her abdomen and on her legs. I am worried.

Monday, August 9, Jean is at home. I phone from work and Roger says he will tell her I called. He says she had tests and her kidneys are "plugged." She canceled lab work for Tuesday and will have it done Wednesday, when she sees a nephrologist.

Tuesday, I talk to Kristin on the phone. She and Roger are trying to get Jean to go outside, as it is a beautiful summer day and Jean loves the outdoors and the sunshine. But she refuses; she is very tired.

Wednesday, I am told at work (the health insurance company where we are both employed, which authorizes all Jean's treatments and manages her health care) that Jean has been admitted to the UConn Health Center Hospital in renal failure. My heart beats fast, and I cry. For days, I have been crying—waves of extreme sadness overcome me unannounced. I am unable to work well, and I stare into space, thinking about when I can next see Jean. After hearing the news of her admission. I leave work quietly in midafternoon and go to the hospital, only 3 miles from work. I watch Jean's room from the hallway for a long time, as doctors and nurses go in and out, closing the door each time they enter or leave. I worry about what is happening, and I watch one doctor run past me down the stairs with tubes of blood. I am sad and scared. Finally I decide to approach a nurse and say I am a friend and ask if it would be appropriate for me to see Jean. I felt so awkward and unsure of myself. I am a nurse by profession, but I feel so humbled and insecure on the other side, being the concerned friend of that nurse's patient. She says she thinks it would be helpful for Jean to see me, as she is "weepy." I said we are all weepy. I quietly enter the room and she is alone, all covered up with only her pink headscarf poking up out of the covers. She looks at me and says, "How did you find me?" "Joan [the oncology case manager at work] told me. Is that okay?" I am afraid she did not want to be found. I am feeling so uneasy and wonder if I am being intrusive. She takes my hand and assures me she is glad to see me. I put my arm around her and tell her to rest, to close her eyes, and we will get the kidneys in order and be on with it for transplant. She obeys like a child and closes her eyes as I soothe her. Her tears fall from beneath closed eyes, and I ache. I tell her to rest and I race back to work, telling no one where I had gone. I had to see her and be sure everything was okay. I cry at my desk.

Thursday, the next day, I go back to the hospital, and look into Jean's room around 2 P.M. She is sound asleep, resting very peacefully. I stand at her bedside and look over her; I want to care for and protect her from pain and hurt. There is now a woman in the bed beside Jean, on the other side of the curtain. The woman looks at me looking longingly and lovingly at Jean and begins to cry. I go to her and I am speechless. We look at each other, and we cry with and for each other. She tells me Jean's "husband" just left. I run down the six flights of stairs and through the lobby and see Roger's car about to pull out of the parking lot. I run after his car like a left-behind puppy. The sweat is running down over my body as I run, and perspiration shows through my blouse. I drive back to work, and go to talk to two close friends of Jean's there, as they wanted to see Jean. I tell them I will be going back to the hospital after work, and one wants to meet me there.

I return to the hospital at 4:30 and enter Jean's room. Kristin and Reid are there; I speak for a minute and leave the room to allow for family privacy. I go stand in the all-too-familiar hallway. Reid joins me and we stand in the hall together, as if on guard. I ask about Kristin and her emotional supports, and he says she has a social worker that she talks to that she and Jean used to see together when Kristin was having some adolescent problems. Reid is a kind young man. He looks unsure of what he is involved in. He answers with short responses and works at making conversation. I study him and feel he is good for Kristin now. He says Kristin had to talk to Jean about a "private matter" and asked him to leave so he wouldn't see her get upset. He later says Jean told Roger she wants to die, and Kristin did not want to hear that kind of talk and was confronting her mother about it. My heart was breaking for a mother and daughter facing life and death together in sorrowful sadness. I waited. Our friend from work came, and I protected the privacy of mother and daughter, saying it was not a good time to go into Jean's room, and she understandingly left. Reid and I waited a very long time.

Kristin came down the hall. She reached for Reid's arms and he comforted her as she cried in deep hurt. I got up and hugged her and she cried so hard. We talked and I tried to comfort her and ease her pain. Tears flowing, she looked at me and said her mother was worried about me—that this was hard on me. We laughed, for that was Jean—always thinking of someone else.

Kristin, Reid, Daren, and Lee—Kristin's and Daren's father and Jean's ex-husband—are going on a long-planned week's vacation; then Kristin will come home for four days and then return to college in Pennsylvania, having been home with her mother all summer. Going on vacation and returning to school are difficult decisions for Kristin. As Kristin and Reid are about to leave, I ask her if she thinks her mom would like to see me. She says yes.

I am so anxious to be with my friend, my confidant, my caregiver for the past 6 years, my teacher, my mentor, my dear, dear friend. I walk into the room; she looks at me and begins to sob like I have never seen Jean cry. I hold her and tell her it's okay. (It's so odd how we say "it's okay" when we are at a loss for something to say when things are not okay.) She tells me she wants to die, and that Kristin and Roger don't want her to. She cries that she wants her family to be with her, and they are going away. She feels helpless and lost. I hold her hand so tight I nearly cut off her circulation. My sweaty, clammy hand tries to make my strength flow to her clenched hand. I stroke her finger lovingly and we talk. I tell her to tell people what *she* wants. She says, "I don't need to see a lot of people, only those who are close to me. I like the peace and quiet. Everything is happening so fast." She cries so hard. "Kristin will be leaving for school, and I know it is best that she go and get on with her life. I am so tired. It takes so much energy to talk to people, to make decisions. I am so tired. I don't know what to do. Dr. Tripp thinks he can help me—more chemo and radiation. What do I do? What if there is a chance and I don't take it? What if something can work?" I say, "Gather the facts—more tests—get the facts and then make a decision. No decision is set in stone." She says, "You mean like start treatment, and then stop?" I say, "Yes. That's an option. Get the facts and make an informed decision." She looks me in the eye and asks, "Will you help me make the decision?" I say, "Yes, I will help you decide."

She tells me of her friend with whom she would sit for 2 hours every night after work 2 years ago. I remember her telling me about going to see her dying friend at that time. I never empathized, or talked to her about it much. I never knew what she was experiencing. Jean goes on to tell me it was so peaceful and quiet and restful and she liked being with her dying friend—a wonderful experience. I say to Jean, then you know what it is like for me to be with you, that I don't want to be anywhere else but with you. She half smiles and understands. Then I say, "But didn't you ever fear you were being intrusive?" She looked me square in the eye and said, almost as if scolding me, "I never worried about being intrusive like you do." Her intonation was telling me I am not intrusive and to stop being such a jerk; I clearly knew what she was saying in so many words, and I knew we would never have to discuss this again. But I did go on: "But you must tell me when enough is enough, and it is time for me to leave." She agrees. And we have an understanding. She reaches for my hand and strokes it, just as I had done hers. She says my hand is cold. I say I am anxious. I tell her my heart is breaking and I feel raw. I get teary, but I don't cry, and her eyes show that she understands my love and concern for her, and probably remembers how she felt 2 years ago with her friend. She tells me she has to use the bathroom and will have to say goodnight; this is a clear cue for me to leave. I hug her and prepare to leave. First I ask her if I can help her to the bathroom, and she makes it clear that she can still walk by herself. She forever portrays a pillar of strength, and there is no self-pity; nor does she want sympathy or pity from anyone else. I leave. [Some time later, she does confide in me that after I left that evening, she did indeed fall, but never told anyone.]

For the first time, I did not cry all the way home [50 miles]. We have an understanding and our ground rules are set. While I was there that evening, Jean's sister, Martha, phoned her. The conversation had been quick; Jean did not want her sister to come to be with her; and now I felt she had decided she wanted me to be with her, as I wanted to be with her. We had talked about the most real, the deepest thing—the choice to live or die, and the decisions she would have to make regarding treatment, and whether I would help with her decisions.

AUGUST 13, 1993

It is Daren's birthday. Jean's mother died on her birthday, a gift, says Jean. Roger's father died on his birthday, a gift, says Jean. Please, no gift for Daren. I go to the hospital at 3 P.M. As I round the hall toward the elevator, I see Roger approaching me. I am confused. He hugs me and says, "Look who is going home!" Behind him in a wheelchair is my dear friend, pink headscarf and cream-colored hat on top of the scarf with a big pink flower on the side of the hat on her head. She is in pink robe and nightgown and her nurse is pushing her in the wheelchair. Roger carries a walker. I do not relate the walker to Jean. In the lobby, while the nurse, Jean, and I wait for Roger to get the car, I tell Jean I am so happy she is going home. Our eyes meet and I wink at her. But at the same time, I am confused—I don't see any medical paraphernalia and I wonder what is up—why home now, in renal failure? For the moment, I don't care. She's going home. I talk to the sweet young nurse: she recognizes me, as I had spoken with her every day when I would go to see Jean. We make small talk, and I think of Jean and me as new Boston University grads so many years ago, not unlike this new young nurse now. I think of all the experiences she has yet to have as a nurse and where she will be 20 years from now, if she will be with a colleague like this. I remember Jean's and my conversation from the night before when I asked Jean if she had received or wanted a backrub, and Jean sarcastically commented on how we learned all these procedures years ago, only for them to become obsolete now. She was a bit angry, even. Anyway, the nurse tells me: "Jean has a rough road ahead." Jean looks up at her and says, nodding toward me, "So does she." I show her a shirt I had just gotten for her with "The Journey" written on it. She has always thanked me for the past 6 years for "being on her journey" with her. She half smiles. Getting into the car is very difficult for Jean. She crawls into the back seat with help from Roger, and very slowly, as if weak and in pain. I want to help, but fumble and am useless. I look into the window and watch as she slowly struggles to get into a comfortable lying-down position in the back seat of his large stationwagon. I want so desperately to help. She finally gets settled, and off they go home, 40 miles away. I leave for the same area, as I must pick up some of my daughter's belongings at UConn on my way home. Once there, I call Roger to see if he needs anything. "No, Kristin has gone to the store to get what supplies we need." I don't tell him I had been sitting in his driveway, before I went to my daughter's dorm, as I had gone directly to the house to help him get Jean out of the car, and up the several several stairs to their raised ranch home. But they were already inside, and I saw no need to disturb their privacy.

I tell him I will be in Storrs (the town where UConn is, 5 miles from their home) on Saturday, and he says to stop by. That is what I wanted to hear, and I say I will call first. Today, Jean is very, very tired, and she can't walk. They will show her how to use the walker. I want to be there with her, as I drive home. Tomorrow, I will see them. For now, I tell Roger I have to see her to tell her "We can handle this," something that Jean always says under all kinds of adverse conditions, and somehow has gotten so many people through crises. Now I want to bounce her words of encouragement back to her. I tell Roger I can take Jean for her first scheduled radiation treatment next Monday. He will tell her. I also plan to tell them I want to spend my upcoming 2 weeks' vacation helping Jean to get back on her feet. I will cancel my trip to Bermuda, a planned vacation with my children to go see their father, who lives there, and instead be with Jean and Roger. They need help, and I need them.

SATURDAY, AUGUST 14, 1993

We need to plan. I call Roger and say I will be by in the morning before I go pick up Erika at UConn to take her home from her prefreshman summer school program. When I arrive, he has gone to get medications, and Kristin is helping Jean in the bathroom. I wait. Jean comes down the hall using the walker. We pile cushions on the couch and set up a mock bed there for her. She sits up for a few minutes, and then tries to get comfortable by lying down, propped with pillows. Roger returns and I say it is time to talk. We can get a commode, a wheelchair, a bed—anything needed, and maybe we should open Jean's case with the VNA. Fortunately, I can have everything ordered and authorized through the oncology case manager who works at the same company where Jean and I work. I had already checked with Joan Grier, the oncology case manager and a mutual friend, in preparation for when the time was right to get supplies ordered. I knew that timing would be important, as I would not want to put anything in place until Jean was ready. She needed to be able to maintain her sense of control. Jean said, "Yes, it is time. We have to develop our resources." I was ready to take action. There was full agreement. I called Joan and she set the wheels in motion for delivery of medical equipment and a VNA visit for the next day.

Roger went to the UConn Health Center to get Jean's medical records for Hartford Hospital, where she was to begin radiation on Monday. Kristin took a bath. I sat on the floor next to Jean as she rested on the couch, and we were finally able to talk privately. She was grateful for getting resources in order, and she made it clear once again she wanted to die sooner rather than later, but Roger and Kristin didn't understand. She said Dr. Tripp (UConn Health Center) felt there was more to be done, and Dr. Carlson (her Hartford Hospital radiologist) would go full speed ahead, too, with radiation. It was hard to read what she *really* wanted. I said, "Maybe Dr. Tripp knows something you don't." There is still hope, but she is so tired. The Ativan doesn't help with sleep; all it does is make her mouth dry. She feels she needs a sleeping pill. I decided not to say anything about my upcoming vacation plans. Roger's brother Lyle and his wife, Claire, were coming up from South Carolina to help out and that would be good for Roger and Jean. I did say that I did not want to go to Bermuda at this time, that I wished someone would tell me to stay home. She said I had to go, but I wondered if she meant it, as when she encouraged Kristin and Daren to go on vacation while wanting them desperately to stay and be with her. Jean dozed, I said good-bye to Kristin, and went home. I called Joan Grier. That night I called Kristin to check in; Jean had told Kristin to ask me to stop by Sunday after Kristin left for school. She was leaving for college in Pennsylvania for the fall semester. I was pleased she asked, and agreed to stop by around lunch time. I felt pleased there was a plan in place for tomorrow, as I knew this was going to be difficult. Now I could sleep. At 3 A.M., I lay awake and wondered what I would say to people—somewhere up the road—if Jean really does die.

SUNDAY, AUGUST 15, 1993

I arrived on schedule. The VNA nurse was giving Jean a bed bath. I met her, but she was not at all communicative. She did her task and left. Roger introduced me as the supervisor from the insurance company that was authorizing payment for her care, but she was not the least bit impressed. I chuckled to myself, as he thought he was making a big and important announcement to her, and she showed absolutely no interest in who was paying for her services, or maybe, I thought, she had no clue about managed care and how all services had to be preauthorized by the insurance company for payment to the VNA. I went in to see Jean—she had taken over Daren's twin bed; she looked beautiful with her aqua gown and turban, and a matching aqua terry robe lying on the chair next to the bed. She had had a bad night, up every 45 minutes to use the bathroom and unable to sleep. She told me cancer patients cannot sleep at night. She was so tired. She had some cornflakes—ate them all. Then Roger went to make himself a sausage sandwich, when I suggested he eat, too, as his stomach was growling loudly. I was going to leave after we had all chatted a bit, and asked Jean if she would like to use the commode before I left. She agreed and we all fumbled with where to put it and how to make it the right height so that Jean could maneuver easily from the bed to it. It was awkward. Finally, after trial placements and much discussion, Jean got to use her new appliance. But always something new to deal with: there was blood in the urine. No panic; we will deal with this, too. We decide to try the wheelchair. We take Jean to the living room in the wheelchair for the first time—she is pleased and says it is comfortable. She sits up and we talk while Roger eats his sandwich, and she has some fresh peaches. I cannot eat, but I am so pleased they are both eating. We do vital signs, which are okay: temp, 98.6°F; pulse, 115; blood pressure, 138 over 96. Roger phones the doctor to report about the blood and is prepared to give vital signs. Jean tires, and we wheel her back to Daren's room and bed. It is already after 2 P.M. Time goes by so fast; routine things like eating and toileting take all day. She is so tired. She thanks me for being there to facilitate transition, as Kristin's leaving today for school is a big change for her and Roger. She wants support for Roger. I feel grateful to be a part of it all, and I look at her, longing for health to return as she falls into a deep sleep.

I go out to talk with Roger. He is hopeful radiation will be done Monday as planned, and for as many treatments as necessary, then more chemo, and then the bone marrow transplant and then remission. I say let's go one day at a time, get the facts tomorrow when she goes to Hartford Hospital to start radiation, and then we go from there. I want to say it has to be Jean's decision ultimately and we cannot jump so far ahead, but I say instead that I want to go with them on Monday. I broach the ambulance topic (Roger has been adamant about driving Jean to her treatment in his car), and I remind him that it is not that he can't do it, but let's see what would be most comfortable for Jean. I imagine that, for him, her having to ride in an ambulance rather than being able to travel in his car must feel threatening, like she is regressing. I suggest, "Let's let her decide." I hug Roger, and he embarrasses me when he says I am a dream come true. I say no, not really, the truth is that I love my friend and I want to help; I really am very selfish. I leave at 3 P.M.

At 8:30 P.M. I phone Roger. Jean had a good sleep and she is up in the wheelchair watching TV in the living room. The blood in the urine is reported to be vaginal, much to her surprise, as the chemo had stopped her menses years ago. I kid her about not getting pregnant now. She ate, she did her routine mouth care, and Roger reports she is doing well. I feel pleased that she is up. The plan is to take two Percocets tonight instead of the Ativan. God, please let her sleep well tonight, as tomorrow will be a very big day.

I am now on vacation for 2 weeks.

The last 2 weeks have seen so many changes day by day. One weekend, we have dinner and sit outside on the back deck. The next weekend we have dinner and Jean is more fatigued and we stay inside so she can lie on the couch. The next day she spends on the couch. One week, she walks me out to the car; the next week she lies on the couch. The third weekend, she is unable to get up unassisted and the house is full of home health appliances. So many changes so fast. Will she now suddenly get better as quickly? Does the pendulum swing both ways? Roger says she is good tonight. Is she? I long to see her tomorrow. When I called tonight, she told Roger to ask me about the ambulance. I told him it was all set. We just had to contact Joan Grier in the morning; I had already prearranged the plan with Joan. Jean is still in charge, and she and I are working together to help Roger accept change. She is a master.

TUESDAY, AUGUST 17, 1993

Today I took Erika and Trevor to the airport for their trip to Bermuda. Yesterday I decided to stay home. Roger and I took Jean via ambulance to Hartford Hospital, where she was seen by Dr. Carlson, her radiologist for the past 9 years, to plan her radiation regime. I ride in the ambulance with Jean, and Roger follows behind in his car. Mark and Darren, the ambulance drivers, chatted freely with Jean and me in the ambulance all the way to Hartford, about 30 miles. While Dr. Carlson examined Jean, I stayed with her, handing her water, raising her head—anything to help her be comfortable, so she could stay in control and concentrate during her conversation with her doctor. She told Dr. Carlson about increasing pressure and discomfort in her abdomen and feeling the tumor growing. She said, "You know I am in renal failure." She understands her illnesss too well. He is gentle and reassuring and will begin full abdominal radiation tomorrow and continue for 4 to 5 weeks. Roger implies she should stay in the hospital. I know she doesn't want to and support the idea of ambulance transfer to and from radiation while she is still well. She will get sicker with nausea and diarrhea later, and maybe then she may need hospitalization. I tell Roger we can do everything at home. She has to be "mapped" for radiation and must lie on her back for 30 minutes—most difficult. She is given morphine to make the test tolerable. Roger and I go for coffee. We force each other to have an English muffin. We go back to Jean and I meet Dr. Raynor, Jean's oncologist, about whom I have heard so much. It is his first day back from vacation and he is truly sorry to see Jean not feeling so well. He has treated her for so many years. He informs Jean that the doctors from UConn Health Center and Hartford Hospital have been in consult already. In the middle of all the talk, Jean has to go to the bathroom. What an ordeal! She is being transported on a stretcher, which doesn't easily fit into the corridors where there is a bathroom. She knows of one bathroom where the stretcher can fit, and she has to direct where to go with exasperation. I suggest we put her onto the ambulance stretcher to avoid extra transfers. We are a team, and as she relates, the small things become so big: going to the bathroom, transferring from a stretcher to the john, for example. I felt so happy to be allowed to stay in the examining room with Jean and Roger and Dr. Carlson. Jean introduced me as her very best friend. It warmed me. She also formally informed Dr. Raynor that Roger and I were her caregivers, and she wanted us with her when he examined and talked with her. Over coffee, I said to Roger I would not go to Bermuda. Later on we would adjust our mutual work schedules so that Jean would not be alone. He agrees.

On our return to Ashford, Jean's home town, I followed the ambulance in Roger's car, bringing Jean's bag with her slippers and hat and an emesis basin I had grabbed at the hospital. Just seeing the room where she had had chemo years ago brought back unpleasant memories and made her nauseated. When we arrived at the house, we were greeted by Roger's brother Lyle and his wife, Claire. Roger and Lyle embraced. Jean commented they had never done that before. Claire hugged Jean and they cried. I went into the kitchen to call Joan Grier to give her the ambulance schedule for the rest of the week so she could authorize the transfers for the insurance coverage. Claire was warm, kind, and honest. She said that the men feel they have to be positive and do not face death. Claire talked openly about it. She was wonderful and Jean is so pleased to have her here. Roger and Lyle went out to fill prescriptions and left the "girls to talk." We did just that. Jean talked about the uncertainty; she explained to Claire that Roger actually believes she will get a bone marrow transplant. We agreed to take one step at a time. The goal of Dr. Carlson right now is to shrink the tumors so the kidneys will function, and Jean will be able to walk without the current pressure on her leg nerves. We agreed a lot had been accomplished today, and we were a good team.

Before he left for the pharmacy, Roger said to me: "See you tomorrow." Jean yelled: "What? She is going to Bermuda." I said: "No, I am not." Jean said we were going to fight. I said she usually won, but not this time. Claire pitched in beautifully and said to Jean, "A vacation is just a change of scenery," and that if I wanted to stay, to accept it, that people are lucky to have one or two extra-special friends. She said nice things, embarrassing me, but made the point that the friendship far surpassed a vacation. Claire said she too could stay as long as needed. We had an honest and productive three-way conversation. I said to Jean, "Never alone" and "One day at a time" and "We can handle this." And I suggested that I go with her tomorrow for radiation, as I now knew where the bathroom was, and Roger could spend time with his family. We all agreed. Jean hugged me tight and long and it was understood that I would be with her, even if she needed to be hospitalized. The days go so fast. I said I would return tomorrow at 10:30. She said, "How about 10:00; come for coffee."

As I drove home, that tremendous wave of sadness hit only once. I had to get Erika and Trevor prepared for their trip to Bermuda. It is good for them to be alone without me, for we never know when we will be forced to be alone. Kristin and Daren are at the New Jersey shore, where Jean and her family used to vacation. Erika and Trevor are going to Bermuda, where we have strong family ties, and where we have always vacationed. As Jean said, "What goes round comes round." She misses Kristin, but is aware she must move on. As she said a few days ago tearfully, "Kristin is letting go, and she needs to." I am glad that Lyle and Claire are with Jean and Roger. I hope she had a good night with her newest medication, a sleeping pill, Restoril, 15 mg.

The kids are en route to Raleigh and then to Bermuda. After I left the airport, I came to Abdows's for breakfast and here I sit writing today's journal, but will soon be on my way to Ashford to continue the journey.

AUGUST 18, 1993

The last two days have been so busy; there is no time to write. It is now midnight and I have just returned home from Ashford.

Yesterday, August 17, I arrived in Ashford around 10:30 A.M. to find Jean sitting up, energetic, and looking terrific. She had slept the night before—the Restoril had worked well. Roger and Lyle had even gone into work in the morning. Jean had some applesauce and we awaited the ambulance to take her for her radiation treatment at Hartford Hospital. She looked so good I could hardly believe it. En route to the hospital, she told me how Claire had pulled up a chair the night before and talked to her about attitude, about being positive and not giving up. She had "lectured" Jean. Anyone else would have turned her off, but Claire had been around and had wisdom and experience, and the talk helped. Jean talked about how wonderful the ambulance ride was compared to riding crumpled up in a car, how she would rather have the ambulance ride than the VNA services if we had to choose between the two for cost-effectiveness in the current managed care environment. I said cost was not the issue, only need was the concern. She wished Hillary Clinton could know how important access to health care is. I marveled to myself as to how worldly and unselfish Jean is to think of Hillary Clinton and the U.S. health care system at such a time when most people would be entirely focused on their own needs and personal crisis. But not Jean. She never ceases to amaze me.

After the first radiation treatment we met with Mary Jane, the oncology nurse in the outpatient cancer center who had worked with Jean through her two former episodes of cancer. We reviewed how to wash the irradiated area, not to use lotions, the importance of nutrition, regular bowel movements, and rest. She kept referring to me when she talked to Jean as "your buddy." I felt like the Buddy Doll recently on the market, but I liked being referred to as Jean's buddy. I found myself worrying about Mary Jane's eye contact toward me as she spoke, rather than directly toward Jean, for I felt Jean was the one she should be addressing. I wondered if Jean noticed, and how it made her feel to have Mary Jane talking so much to her buddy instead of to her, the patient. Jean went on to explain her concerns about the Ensure nutrition supplement she was currently using: it had so much potassium, and her potassium level was already elevated due to kidney failure. Mary Jane arranged for Ann, the dietitian, to call Roger. We were also told blood work would be done two times a week, as the creatinine level (a measure of kidney function) was high. I asked about a prescription for Compazine for nausea and we were to call the doctor, if needed. It was a successful treatment stay at Hartford Hospital. On the way home, Jean dozed on and off. At one point she said, "You really should write a book, Linda. There is so much involved. Every day is different; there is always something new to deal with. So much energy is needed. You never know what will be dealt to you next."

Jean had asked Jane, her friend and former social worker–therapist who had worked with her and her daughter a few years ago, to come by this evening. Jean said I could stay and meet her. I said I would play it by ear, that I would love to meet her, but I was unsure as to whether it would be appropriate for me to stay for the session. Jean said she told Roger that Claire and Lyle could join in as well. She asked me whose call it should be who should be there for the therapy session. I said both she and Roger should discuss it, but that it was ultimately really her decision; I suggested she talk to Roger when we get home. When we arrived at the house, I said to Roger that Jean wanted to plan for the 4 P.M. meeting with Joyce; Roger said he could not be there, that he had another appointment. I decided I had best leave. I told Roger I would like to come back tomorrow for the second treatment, unless he preferred to go himself. He said he would be happy to have me go again. I asked Claire if she minded, or if she wanted to go instead of me. She said that she had gotten a lot done at the house while we were gone, but would go if I was unable. I left around 3:30 P.M. No tears on the way home. My long-time home-town friend, Joyce T, called and invited me over to dinner. I went for a run and then to Joyce's, though I truly would rather have stayed home with my journal. Intellectually, I knew I needed to balance myself and forced myself to go and refocus for a while. We had a nice dinner, but all I wanted to talk about was Jean, as everything else seemed so trivial. On the way home, I stopped at CVS to get Jean some Neutrogena soap, one of the kinds recommended for her irradiated skin. They were on sale, three bars for the price of two. I knew Jean would be pleased with a bargain!

Something I nearly forgot to mention: On my way home from Jean's house, I phoned work to let the people know that Jean was progressing with treatments, family was with her, and she was working to conserve energy. So many well-meaning friends and coworkers were calling Roger for updates on Jean, and he was tiring, too. I suggested I would be in touch regularly, and anyone could call me if they wanted to. They were pleased to hear about their friend and sent their love and prayers to Jean and family. I promised to notify them of any change. Jean had helped so many people through the years with their personal crises, and had always been available to anyone. People were missing her, and I knew that. I also knew how lucky I was to be with her daily. I did not take the honor for granted.

When I got home from dinner at Joyce's, I phoned Joan Grier and asked her to order a hospital bed and told her that the geri-chair had been returned for a motorized recliner. We talked about confidentiality and that Jean had agreed that Joan and I would manage Jean's care. (Employees of the insurance company can choose not to have their care managed at all because of the confidentiality issue; other employees would have access to a peer's medical care.) My role was becoming more clearly defined: caregiver and case manager. I went to sleep at 10:30 P.M. and slept through the night for the first time in many nights.

WEDNESDAY, AUGUST 18

Today when I arrived at Jean's home, Jean was in her new hospital bed. She could manage the controls and was much more comfortable. This was good timing once again. The ambulance was late, which caused some tension, but we were finally off close to schedule. During the ambulance ride into Hartford, Jean again commented on how much easier it was to ride via ambulance. She was now experiencing a fair amount of pain and was taking Percocet, 10 mg every 4 hours. It was 2 P.M. and the noon dose had just started to work; I felt concerned that the pain med was not being very effective. Fortunately, the ride was comfortable. We talked. Jean had been napping when Jane, her social worker and friend, called the house to come over as planned. Roger told Jane that Jean was sleeping and did not offer to wake her, so Jane did not come over. Jean was very upset when she awoke. Roger called and made an appointment for the next day. Jean and Roger had had a pretty serious argument, but it was a sign of progress that Roger did call to make another appointment. The conflict took so much of Jean's energy. She feels so strongly that Roger needs to talk and face things as they are. I said that events of last night were part of the process, and there was progress.

We made it for the second radiation treatment. I watched the treatment on the monitor in the office outside the treatment room. My poor dear friend. She had shown me her abdomen earlier today and I had felt the nodes so close to the surface of the skin. They were mostly on the right side, and her right leg was so sore and swollen. I felt her ankle; there was pitting edema and I ached inside. Her abdomen was marked, and I watched the monitor, observing where the radiation had to hit. I hoped she did not hurt lying on that hard table and I felt like I wanted to be in there with her, for I did not want her to be alone, even for the radiation. I felt like the pet dog waiting for its master longingly and anxiously. Once the treatment was done, she was wheeled out on the stretcher, and I directed us to get the lab work done. I had already spoken to Mary Jane, who notified the lab nurse and Ann, the dietitian, that we needed to see them as well as Dr. Raynor while we were at the hospital.

Blood was drawn. Ann came to explain about the new supplement, Suplena, low in potassium. And finally Dr. Raynor came into the examining room where we were waiting. Jean informed him of her pain and swelling in the leg, about diminished urine output. She was drowsy and I helped with the rest of the things she wanted to tell Dr. Raynor. He talked about going to a patch, Duragesic 25 mg, for pain, and he wrote the prescription. The serious underlying questions are not asked. For now, we look for relief and radiation to shrink the nodes. Staff at the center all know Jean and stop by continually to say hello. She brightens when she sees them, and I know she musters the energy from the depth of her toes to talk to them all. We have everything done in an hour. I have the prescription, the supplement, the water bottle (Jean always has a bottle of ice water, as her mouth gets so dry), my nurse's notes, and my best friend— and off we go to Ashford.

Jean raises her legs for comfort on the stretcher in the ambulance, securing her feet in the ties on the stretcher. We talk about NU 101 (a Fundamentals of Nursing course that all nursing students at BU took), and I comment on how much we actually learned, how much we were taught and didn't forget, body alignment included. She dozes, and I keep my hand touching her leg, as if I was keeping her on the stretcher over bumps and curves, always with a watchful eye on her. She looks up and asks if I got my kids off to Bermuda okay. I assure her I did, yesterday. She asks, "How was it?" I said, "It was wonderful." She said it was wonderful for her and for Roger that I stayed. "This is where I want to be." I was so happy that she said what she did. I told her that I felt I needed to clarify with Kristin why I stayed behind, and that Kristin had made the right decision to go on her vacation a few weeks back.

I told Jean we would write a book. We had enough material; there is so much to tell. We would call it "Friends' Journey." The ambulance driver asked if we went to nursing school together. I said, "Yes, to BU," and we conversed more about it. It felt like Jean and I went way back, though we never knew each other during those nursing school days. I told him we had probably passed each other in the halls, never to know we would one day work together; never to know we would one day be riding in an ambulance together under such conditions; Jean smiled. We also talked about our frequent commute back and forth to work along Route 84, and now by ambulance for very different reasons.

When we arrived home, Jean sat in her new recliner, and we three women talked while Roger and Lyle went to fill the prescription for the Duragesic patch. Jean phoned the pharmacy herself to order the Suplena supplement. I was surprised to see her take charge as in the old days. She spoke slowly and assertively, and I loved watching and listening to her on the phone. My mind flashed back to the many years of listening to her on the phone at work. I enjoyed this moment and again marveled at my wonderful friend.

Jean drank two-thirds of a can of Suplena and then rested. Before our dinner, she retired to her new hospital bed. An hour later, she called me into her room. She was shaking and very tremulous. The air conditioner was on high and she asked for two more quilts. She asked me what to do. She was panicked. I helped her with deep, slow breaths. Slowly she regained her composure. I took her temperature: 100.2°F. We forced ice water, lowered the air conditioner, removed covers. Her next temperature was 101.2°F. We continued to take off covers and push ice water. Finally, after 2 hours, her temp came back down to 100.2°F. As I sat with her, she asked about my writing—logging, she called it. I said that the writing helps, and I am reading as well, books about coping, and commented she had taught me well about journaling. Again I said we would write this story together. In time as she started to feel better, I would share this journal with her, and she could add, from her perspective. I asked her what she had done with her journal she had kept over the years. She said she was sorry; she had destroyed it just days ago when she cleaned out material she did not want to leave behind. She cried (one of the last times I would see her cry this much) and said she was sorry. She did not know that anyone would want it and now realized that, of course, I would. But when she had reread it only a few days before, it was so painful she threw it away. I felt bad because I had wanted her writing to keep forever— something so personally hers to become a part of me. Tears filled my eyes as well, but I told her it was good that she had thrown it away because it was painful. We have plenty to write now anyway. She asked what I wrote about. I said, "Everything. I can hardly believe there is so much to write about." I told her it would be our story and asked her if she wanted to be referred to as Jean Elisabeth or Jean E. She asked me what I thought, and I said that I was really a follower at heart, and that she should decide. She said: "Linda Q. and Jean E." She cried and said, "Would you please write the story, even if I am not here?" I said it would be our story and our names would be together. I went on to promise that I would share what I was writing with her as she started to feel better, and we would talk more about it, but that now she needed to rest. She looked so lovingly at me and said this must be difficult for me. I said that she gives me strength. She asked if I had read "Transitions." I said I was reading it. A special friend, Charlie, former CEO of our company, had given it to her a few years ago. I didn't tell her I was also reading the Sloan-Kettering rabbi's book on grief and loss. I felt like crying. She asked if there were something I needed to talk about. I said, "No, we would talk later." I felt she needed to rest. But I think now that maybe I am being like Roger, and maybe I need to talk to Jean about my sadness, too. I didn't know. I wished my friend Ed, a psychologist, were available to advise me. I wished I could sit in with Jean's therapist, Jane. I don't know what is right.

After Jean used the commode, she had severe pain in her leg. At first I felt helpless, but then I thought and reminded her that lying on her back had been comfortable before. She changed position to lie on her back, and it helped. She later commented on how nursing is so important. I had removed the covers when she was hot, told her to take off her turban when her temp went up, kept making her drink ice water, and now reminded her how to lie comfortably. I didn't want to leave. Roger invited me to stay the night. I said I will stay some evening, but tonight I would go home. I kissed my friend so gently and said I would return tomorrow. She thanked me.

Earlier, Peter, Paul, and Mary were in concert on the TV in the living room, and we all listened. Most of the time, I sat near Jean in her bedroom and listened with her as we could hear them on the TV in the living room. She commented on how special it was for all of us to be together—Roger, Claire, Lyle, me, and her, listening to Peter, Paul, and Mary, favorite folk singers from the 1960s and 1970s. I agreed and said I would not want to spend my vacation any other way; it seemed we were momentarily all at peace. She thanked me again for staying home from Bermuda. The songs were perfect: "I'll walk by your side in the the rain." She is so beautiful, my friend, Jean E., and I'll stay by her side forever.

FRIDAY, AUGUST 20, 1993

On Thursday, August 19, at 8:30 A.M., Roger called to say the hospital had called him and that Jean's creatinine level had risen to 6. Jean would be admitted today to Hartford Hospital, but he had not yet told her. I knew this would be a blow to Jean as she so desired to be at home, and I, too, so wanted her to be able to stay home, as she desired. It was a beautiful sunny day and I was anxious to get to Ashford, but delayed going until late morning. When I got into the car, I began to cry, and as I drove I told myself I could only cry until a certain distance and then must stop. I thought a lot about crying, that it is an expression and release, but enough is enough—it would not change anything and would be self-defeating if carried to an extreme. I thought about Rabbi Pesash's book on grief and loss. He writes that getting lost in despair robs you of life, which is such a precious gift. The tears flowed so freely and I knew that to get by Baker's Restaurant without extreme sadness would be impossible. Jean and I had met there for breakfast a few times these past 6 months during her chemotherapy. By the time I reached the restaurant, I had been crying for 12 miles. I took a deep breath as I passed. Then I drove on to the Route 84 intersection, another 6 miles, where I opened the windows, breathed the fresh air, and forced a smile to rid my face of the sadness I felt. I wanted to be up and positive when I reached the house, another 12 miles away.

When I arrived, Claire and Jean were talking in the bedroom; Claire had just told her the facts—that her creatinine level was elevated and she would be going into the hospital. Jean had rested well in the morning and looked refreshed. She said she had had a wash with Roger's help earlier, and she would agree to home health aides from now on! We laughed. She was in light blue, turban and all, and looked so pretty to me. It felt good to be with her and away from my sadness all the way over. While Jean dozed, I sat in the chair in her room and closed my eyes, too. I was pleased to be quiet in her restful company. In time, she suggested a trip to the bathroom, and I lifted her out of bed to the wheelchair without Roger's help for the first time—with her permission, of course, as she called all the shots and directed all the movements of those who assisted her, always in control. I could lift her and help her mobilize without anyone else's assistance; this was important for me to know, and the knowledge that Jean and I could mobilize on our own offered a sense of security. She went to her new recliner chair, and we all sat around talking as we waited for the ambulance to take Jean to the hospital. I charted the medications, Roger packed the suitcase, Claire prepared the water bottle—we all had our roles and tasks. Jean looked comfortable in her recliner chair in a cozy black and white wrap, which the staff of our department at work had given her.

The ambulance arrived on time, and the driver was the same person who had come the past 3 days. He was becoming familiar and, at this time, a bit too personal. But we handled his somewhat intrusive questions well, abruptly, but not rudely, so he got the picture and retreated. On the other hand, Jean commented that the consistency of having the same driver was nice, as he knew where to go into the house, which steps to pay particular attention to, how the door opened, etc. Not having to explain the nuances to a new driver each time and wondering if he was going to be able to execute the process of lifting and carrying the stretcher down multiple flights of stairs meant Jean expended much less energy and felt more secure.

And we were definitely in a conservation-of-energy mode, as medications, radiation, and kidney problems were all taking a toll on Jean's diminishing energy.

On the ambulance ride to the hospital, Jean looked so alert and rested. She was not in pain and was actually comfortable. The Duragesic patch was working. Roger followed us in the car. I hoped I was not usurping his place by riding in the ambulance. Through the window, I could see him smoking a cigarette as he drove behind the ambulance, and I was uncertain of his expression, which I tried unsuccessfully to read. I waved and he waved back. At the hospital, we transferred her from the stretcher to the radiation table like an experienced team. I took her head, adjusting pillows so she would land perfectly. I was also now diligently watching body alignment, as I knew that how she lay these days was vital to comfort, and the pain medication would mask uncomfortable positioning only temporarily.

From radiation, we went directly to Center-11, the oncology unit, for admission. The room was beautiful, and the unit was quiet. A nurse came in to see Jean, and I introduced myself as Jean's case manager. She was not impressed and had nothing to say to me. Jean smiled and spoke to all her old friends on the staff of C-11. Dr. Rayner came in and I motioned to Jean, "Should I leave?" She shook her head "no," and I stayed. He had consulted with Dr. Carlson, the Hartford Hospital oncology radiologist, Dr. Carlyle, the nephrologist, and all the doctors involved at UConn Health Center, and all were in agreement that a stent, or artificial tube, should be placed in the kidney to assist with urine flow to the bladder.

Dr. Carlyle, the nephrologist, entered the room and began his litany of how he would not recommend surgery if there was nothing else that could be done, but that in Jean's case, there was consensus that treatment could still be done. He talked, on the other hand, about death from kidney failure being not unpleasant—that people in kidney failure just "fall asleep and pass." Roger introjected strongly that we are positive, that he and Jean know all this, that they had led a cancer support group for 6 years. He was angry, for he did not want to hear any reference to giving up or death. I felt that Dr. Carlyle was leading to the positive position that in Jean's case there was hope for further treatment, but for those for whom there is no hope, death by kidney failure is not physically painful. Roger and I just heard the same thing differently, illustrating that perception is everything in communication.

On the heels of Dr. Carlyle came Dr. Stalkner, the urologist. He, like Dr. Carlyle, was young. As Dr. Carlyle left, Jean thanked him for his directness. Dr. Stalkner had a warmer affect as he took the spotlight. He shook hands with both Roger and me, acknowledging our presence, unlike Dr. Carlyle. He explained the procedure of placing a stent into the tubes leading from the kidneys. He talked about all the possibilities of entering the stent from the top or from the bottom, or actually having to do a nephrostomy, where the tubes exist through the back. After he left, Jean turned to me and said, "Do you believe these doctors—their direct manner, good eye contact, informative explanations?" We agreed we were both impressed with their training and marveled at how young they were! Jean, God love her, had asked, "How about surgery tonight; why wait until morning?" Dr. Stalkner said he would prefer to do it with the "first team" of staff, who work on the day shift. That made good sense to us, though I know Jean was thinking of it being more cost-effective to do the surgery right away rather than waste a possible extra day in the hospital. This is exactly how she used to manage care at work, insisting that treatment begin immediately upon admission!

Debbie, the nurse, came in and took yet another medical history from Jean, asking many redundant questions that had already been answered in previous interviews. She was not warm and definitely not in tune with the needs of the anxious cancer patient and family members. She had to get her tasks done, without even recognizing the person she was interviewing. She was not empathetic toward Jean and her obvious extreme fatigue after all she had been through already today. The Duragesic patch had fallen off, for instance, but that was of no concern to this nurse. She then inserted a rectal suppository into Jean, but had neglected to get a commode. Her priorities were all messed up, and I was angry; this woman shared my profession and made it look so bad. I went out to the nurse's station and asked others for a commode—didn't anyone recognize how important it was for Jean to have a commode, so she would not mess herself? I was terribly annoyed. Didn't they realize how uncomfortable it would be for her to even try to sit on a bedpan because of her pain, that she had not had a bowel movement for 5 days? Where was the commode? I would get it! Finally after telling four different individuals of our need for a commode, I found an aide who helped me bring one to Jean's bedside.

Roger, Jean, and I talked about relationships; I had no brothers or sisters, but I talked about how you can at least choose your friends. Roger talked about a friend and coworker who called him "Dad," as hers had passed away and she had become very attached to Roger as a father figure. And Roger and Jean agreed they had both adopted family along the way in their lives; this woman was his adopted daughter, not hers, and she respected that. We agreed Jean could be my sister.

Dr. Fay, the handsome psychiatrist Jean had seen several times in the past 6 months on the oncology unit, walked in next. Again I suggested I leave, but he motioned me to stay. He talked with Jean about "where she was" now, and I wondered how different she might look to him now, as he had not seen her in several weeks. She talked about the procedure to be done and alluded to some of their past therapy work on "when to call it," as far as treatment goes. He said, "And where will that come from?" "Me," she said. And he said, "From where?" I did not understand and neither did Jean. He said he would probably not see her again while she was in the hospital, but to call him when the radiation treatments were done. She was very fatigued. He asked her if she made mistakes mentally, or if things were slipping by her. I had said she had a "Daracef" patch on. Only Dr. Fay picked up on the error, that it was a "Duragesic" patch. He thought it odd that no one else noticed the mistake, particularly Jean, who is generally quick to pick up on such errors. He asked if that happened often now. He seemed to be noticing something. I assured him that Jean's mental status was good, that nothing got by her usually, and that she was fully aware. Later I was in the hallway, and he approached me and said that he had asked about Jean's mental status because he noticed a clear change in Jean. He said she does not follow a thought and drifts as if she has a hidden, or unspoken, fear. He correlated that possibly with the anxiety reaction she had had. I felt incompetent—that maybe I was missing something—but I wanted to assure him her mentation was okay, that she spoke of life-and-death issues often with me, but it was difficult with Roger and Kristin. In the room, he had said that each person's different perspective was good. I suggested he could help us all with this issue. He smiled handsomely. Next entered the anestheseologist, and by now the questions were very tiring, so I began to answer for Jean to help conserve some of her dwindling energy after such a day.

SATURDAY, AUGUST 21

It has been so busy that I must write now for the past two days.

Friday, August 20: Jean was scheduled for surgery to have the stents put in at 1:45 P.M. In the morning, I called the insurance company [our employer] to clarify that I would manage Jean's care, as she had asked me to be her case manager officially. As there was confusion and difficulty in the transition of her care to me from the usual medical case manager, I decided to go in early to speak with the staff at the Hartford Hospital oncology unit. Just as I arrived on Center-11, Jean was being placed on a stretcher to be taken to the OR. She saw me, and said, "Hi, love!" I was confused as she was not scheduled for surgery for hours yet, but I escorted her to the elevator and asked the attendant if I could go with her to the OR. Initially, I was told no, but I insisted, and with a little persistance and special permission, I was allowed to go. (Generally only parents of young children are allowed to go down to the OR waiting area.) Jean told me Dr. Carlson had seen her earlier and she had asked him for honesty. He told her that it was difficult for him as she was so special. She cried as she told me, and I hugged her as she lay on the stretcher awaiting the elevator. She had a look in her eye that she knew things were progressing rapidly downhill. I focused her on the impending surgery, and how this was a positive step and to take this one step at a time. She agreed. We sat in the OR waiting room a long time. She was in no pain. She looked at me and said: "Isn't it strange how we always come together?" I said, "Yes, there certainly was a power far stronger than us." It was fate that I arrived just as she was going to the OR earlier than scheduled and Roger was not yet there. She would have been alone had I not coincidentally appeared. After she was taken to the OR, I went upstairs and met with her primary nurse on Center-11. I tried to clarify that I would be the case manager from our insurance company from now on, coordinating Jean's care to keep it simple and consistent and to allow Jean to conserve her energy. She said Jean had already told her I would coordinate her care, but she had not yet told the hospital medical case manager who normally manages the care of clients for our insurance company. I explained I had already spoken to that nurse as well, and then I went on to explain my total involvement in Jean's care and my commitment to her and her family. She gave me positive feedback for caring for my friend. Then I sat with Roger, who had arrived after Jean was taken to the OR, and we waited for the outcome of the surgery. After one and a half hours, the urologist called Roger, and Roger asked me to speak with him. The operation had been a success; the stents were in place, though with difficulty; He had used the biggest size stent he could; the kidneys looked normal, and he hoped that they would not clog and renal function would return. Roger and I hugged and cried tears of relief. Roger waited for Jean to be returned to her room, and then he left for home. I said I would stick around and then leave after I felt all was okay. I stayed by Jean's bedside. Later the urologist who performed the surgery came by. The stents were not draining. He irrigated them and still no return. He told Jean; she was semiconscious, probably stuporous from the anesthesia. After he left, I checked her drainage tubes again, and she looked at me and said, "Not working." I explained what the doctor had said, and that a second procedure would have to be done—plan B. I waited all night. Roger beeped me. I called him to let him know I would inform him as soon as they decided to reoperate. Finally, at 11:30 P.M. the OR called for Jean to return for a nephrostomy tube implant. I called Roger and he said he would be right in. Again, they took Jean to the OR before Roger got there; again I accompanied her, being as positive as I could. Roger arrived after they had taken her into the radiology room where they would do the procedure, and we sat and waited. At 12:30 A.M., the radiologist appeared. They had been unable to place the tubes; they would not hold in the kidneys. The diagnosis was "nonobstrustive renal failure." We went back to the room. Jean looked frightened and very weary. I sat outside her room and wept. Roger told me Jean wanted to see me. I entered with red eyes, and she said we would now all need Kleenex. It had been such a trying day.

After the first surgery, I had watched over her. Because she had presented as more groggy and confused, I had called staff, who ordered a blood check. Sure enough, the creatinine level had risen to 7. I told them they had to do a second procedure tonight. I had watched over Jean all day and night, and now two surgical procedures had failed in one day. I feared my friend would die of kidney failure. Roger and I stayed all night, sleeping in chairs, one on each side of Jean's bed. Jean must have thought we were gathered because she was surely dying. I explained that this was not the case. I dozed lightly on and off. At dawn, Jean awoke and announced: "I am still alive. I didn't die!" She made me smile. The plan for the day was for Roger and me to go home and Claire and Lyle to come in. I would return in the afternoon and Roger would return in the evening.

I raced home and lay down after 24 hours without sleep. The phone rang four times. I got up, showered, and decided to head back to Hartford [a 50-mile trip]. Roger beeped me that James, Jean's brother from New York, was driving up to see Jean. I was anxious to meet James, whom Jean had spoken about so tenderly. When I arrived at the hospital, Claire and Lyle were anxious to tell me that the doctors and Jean had decided against dialysis. The concern now was that Roger accept this decision. The plan was for the doctor to call Roger and for Lyle to talk with Roger about the decision. I hoped Roger would be in agreement.

I went in to see Jean. She was asleep, so I just sat and watched her chest rise and fall with deep, slow breaths. In walked a tall, handsome, well-dressed man. I said, "Hello, James." I introduced myself. He looked intently at Jean as she slept, and he looked surprised. Asleep, I am sure she looked comatose to him. I got up and gently wakened her. "Look, Jean. Look who is here." She slowly opened her eyes and immediately beamed when she saw James and his daughter Sara. I left the room and heard her telling James all about me, how I canceled my trip to Bermuda to be with her, how we had gone to BU together, worked together, and about my children even. On and on she went about me, and I felt a little embarrassed. I left them alone for quite a while. After some time, I quietly reentered as I expected it would be awkward for James, not knowing Jean's needs, which were becoming many: having her water always available so she could keep her mouth wet to be able to talk, keeping her head raised at just the right height so she could be as comfortable as possible, helping with her train of thought, which could wander. We all four chatted, and Jean kept up beautifully. She was quick and humorous and stayed with the conversation. It was wonderful. I loved meeting James, the male version of Jean; they were so much alike. I told him so, and he accepted my comments as a compliment. We were instant friends.

Later James came into the hall with me as Sara stayed with Jean. He talked about very personal family matters, about issues with their other sister and her wanting to be a part of the planning of the memorial service, for example. He gave me all his phone numbers where he could be reached 24 hours a day and took my phone and beeper numbers. We were comforted to have each other's numbers for immediate access to one another. He thanked me and I explained that I loved his sister and she was most special to me, that she had touched my life like no one else had, and his eyes teared. I asked him if he ever had a close friend ill like this, and he said he didn't have any close friends. I thought it odd, for he was so kind, warm, gentle, and honest. He had told Jean to make her own decision about dialysis, regardless of pressure from anyone else, to follow her own heart. He said to her, as she had said to him so many times during his recent personal crisis, "Trust through the panic." He said how much Jean had helped him during his emotional problems, and I said she had helped so many people, but he was always her first and foremost priority. He remembered talking to me on the phone at work when he had tried to call Jean and she was unavailable, and Jean explained to him how I had been instructed by her to call her whenever he called no matter where she was or what she was doing. We chuckled about how Jean abused company time only this once. I liked James and felt immediately connected; that was good, as I was beginning to realize the inevitable might happen. Roger came in; he had been crying. James left and I said I would see him soon, if he were going to visit again. I did not mean to imply "when Jean dies." He understood and we agreed we would see what happens. I felt he would call me often over the next few weeks. I hoped so. Roger and Jean talked and then Roger came out into the hall to get me. It was agreed—no dialysis; I knew this was terribly difficult for Roger, but he had finally agreed. The plan was to continue on with the radiation until Dr. Carlson said to stop. We were all in agreement. Roger cried. My friend looked relieved that the issue had been settled and there was resolution. The intravenous was discontinued. Jean was told by staff that she could now eat what she wanted. Jean commented that for years she had been counting this and that food ingredient, watching her potassium intake like a hawk the past few weeks, and other things too numerous to mention—and then they tell you will die and you can have anything! "I could eat custard every day for the rest of my life," she said, and punctuated the comment with a sarcastic laugh.

The Foley catheter from the bladder drained twice as much today as it did yesterday. Could the kidneys be picking up in function? Creatinine 7, BUN 120. I suggested there may be hope for better kidney function. I also told Jean she was a blessed woman because now she was no longer in pain, as she had been. She noticed and agreed.

I would leave for today, but would return tomorrow, Sunday, as Kristin would be arriving after a week's vacation with her father and brother. I cried hard all the way to Vernon, halfway home. It struck me suddenly how an hour before at the hospital, I had fed my beautiful, tall, elegant, dignified friend her dinner for the first time. It tormented me—the thought that I now had to feed her, that she was that ill and weak. But she had so elegantly transitioned me to this new task. She had instructed me so cleverly, making the transition natural and easy. Sara, James's daughter had tried to feed Jean some Jell-O, and it was difficult and awkward for both. Jean had suggested that I help, and I obediently took over. At first, feeling clumsy, I slowly spooned the Jell-O to her mouth; after a few bites, I was in step with Jean and she maintained her dignity, ordering me as to what food item from the tray to feed in what sequence. I had to concentrate so much on the process she designed that I forgot the uneasiness involved with feeding one's friend and colleague. We developed an easy rhythm, and her dinner was all eaten. My love for her was growing daily. But the fact that she was so ill that I now had to feed her hit me hard in Vernon. I stopped and phoned Joan Grier, my friend at work who was also following Jean's care, and I spoke with her of my overwhelming sorrow. She provided support; I felt better to have talked to someone and drove the rest of the way home.

SUNDAY, AUGUST 22

I awoke to realize that today would have been my father's 75th birthday. I would not tell Jean, for she believes it is a gift for a loved one to die on another's birthday. I got to Hartford Hospital in time to enter with the 7 A.M. shift, two coffees in hand, one for Roger, one for me. As I got off the elevator on Center-11, I met Roger going for a coffee. We talked and he reported he had turned Jean frequently during the night, and tended to her needs for drink and toileting. He had not gotten to sleep until 4 A.M. He asked me to call him after Dr. Carlson came in on his morning rounds, as he was going to go home and get some needed and well-deserved rest. I went in to see my friend. She looked rested, alert, and so happy to see me. I was clearly happy to see her. I noticed the Foley catheter was draining better. I finally settled down to relax and just simply be with her while she rested. Then breakfast arrived. I set the tray before her and remembered feeding her her last evening meal and wondered what to do now. Was she more rested? Would she want to try to feed herself now? Was she embarrassed? What to do. She then commented on my taking over feeding her last night from Sara, and that it was positive. I said it must seem awkward to her, but that it really was just another point on the continuum of care, and that it felt so natural for me to do—I loved feeding her and it was okay. I let her choose what to eat; she wanted brown sugar for her cream of wheat. I immediately went to ask for some, as there was none on the tray. The aide would try to get some. In the meatime, we used white sugar quite successfully. I fed her gently but assertively. It was so comfortable and natural to provide nourishment for my sick friend. She maintained her dignity and I felt humbled by the privilege of feeding such a strong, magnificent woman. I told her she taught me so much each day. I thought to myself (as always) what a master and teacher she is and how small I always feel in her presence. My love for her was growing more and more each day and I cherished this moment with her. I knew that from this point forward we need not discuss the feeding issue again, that it was understood that I would feed her from now on. We had understanding.

After breakfast, Lyle and Claire walked in. I felt disappointed to have our private moment interrupted, and I hoped the expression on my face did not reveal my dismay.

I explained that Jean had expected Lee (her former husband and father of her children) to come in, and she needed to get a bath and get ready for his visit. Earlier Jean had felt a need to speak with Lee and I had phoned him for her, as she had requested. She spoke to him on the phone and asked him to come see her. Kristin and Daren would be coming, too. As we talked, Jean's sister Martha and husband, Bill, appeared from nowhere. I went into the hallway and Martha introduced herself, saying James had fallen in love with me immediately; she informed me she was prepared to stay for as long as need be with Jean. She was going to take over. Somehow, I got in to Jean to tell her that Martha was planning to stay. I wanted to warn and prepare Jean, as I knew this would be trying for her to handle. She loved her sister, but they had very different personalities. Martha was very pressured in her affect, and Jean needed a quieter, gentler approach at this time; and she needed to continue to feel in control. She did not want Martha to take over. Jean had talked about all this. (She had told me weeks earlier that she cannot tolerate people with high energy around her when she is feeling weak and tired. She had very good friends that she would not even see because of this intolerance, which in no way diminished her love or concern for them.) I then left the room while the family spoke together. Eventually, I went toward the door so Jean could catch my eye. I stood where only Jean could see me outside her doorway. Finally, she clarified with Martha that Roger and Linda are caring for her. I heard "Linda this" and "Linda that," and I knew that was my cue to reenter. I knew Jean well enough to read her cues. As I entered, Jean said to me that they were chatting about her care plan, giving me the opening to validate. I chirped in that it was all set and plans were in place. I had already spoken to Claire about what Jean wanted as far as care goes, that she wanted us all to continue as we were doing. At this point, Claire took charge and assertively suggested that she and Lyle and Martha and Bill go to the cafeteria for coffee, so that Jean could get her bath. It was not easy, but Claire finally got her message across and her mission was accomplished. Jean and I were once again left alone to get Jean ready for Lee's arrival. Before all this had transpired with Claire, Martha had commented on how Jean was going to a better place with God, etc. As she was speaking, Jean had turned to me, sitting close by her left side, and said: "Isn't she a trip? She's very religious." Martha was continuing to talk in very religious ways. I whispered to Jean: "You're a love," and winked at her, she had tickled me with her quiet comment while her sister was going on and on about heavenly things in her own supportive way.

I got the nurse and together we helped Jean get ready for Lee and her children to visit. She had a bath and I watched to learn—to refresh my nursing skills so that in the near future I could take over completely, as I knew I eventually would. I asked Jean's permission, of course, to be part of such a private ceremony and watched as the nurse used so many washcloths and gloves to bathe her beautiful and elegant body. In my day as a bedside nurse, we never used such a multitude of towels and never wore gloves. I tried to honor Jean's privacy and looked away except when she was covered, for I did not want to embarrass her. Earlier, she had instructed me to check her catheter when it felt uncomfortable and we thought she may have pulled on it. We were continuing the transition to full care, but ever so gently and gingerly. I helped make the bed and chose a pretty pink spread to match Jean's lovely pink nightwear and turban. She looked ravishing, and before Lee came, she asked if she should put on some lipstick. I said something like, "Be real, no way!" She agreed: "What for?" She looked so pretty; she did not need lipstick. As her bath was finishing, Lee walked in. I escorted him out to the hall and we chatted. He remembered me from 5 years ago, when I spoke at a convention of mental health providers at the Marriott Hotel. He thanked me for helping Jean, and I said, "No thank you's are necessary. Jean is very special to me, and it is a privilege to be with her." I said that he and Jean must also have a very special relationship. He agreed; after all, neither he nor she had ever remarried, and he felt that said something of their relationship. He went in to see Jean, and I went to go find Lyle and Claire.

I could not find them, so I decided to go see the hospital chapel. It was all blue and quiet and peaceful, and I was alone with my thoughts. I didn't quite know what to do, where to sit or stand, so I leaned against the back wall and tried to pray. But all I could do was cry. I felt so wounded and sad, and with the tears, I prayed for my friend, that she never feel pain and die a beautiful death. I thought about how I, too, could now accept death, for I would once again be with her upon my own death. It was a comforting thought, and I thought about how she and I should talk about death and what it means to her and to me.

Earlier, when the aide had taken her blood pressure, Jean asked if it went down or up as you were dying. He didn't respond. After he left, she also made me take her pressure again, as she felt he had not done it right. I felt honored to be asked to do this task, that she trusted me above the others. And I knew I would satisfy that trust and her faith in me. I felt empowered to take care of her every need from bath to blood pressure. She told me she did not know how to die; she had never seen someone die before. I was surprised, and then I realized I had never seen someone die, either. I had seen dead bodies, but had never been with someone dying all the way. I said we live and we are not told how to live; we die as we live—a natural process. I asked if she was afraid. I said I was not afraid—we would go through this together. And then someone interrupted us. We were forever being interrupted.

After I left the chapel, I returned to Jean's room, and she beamed when I entered. Lee had left. I asked how she was. I gave her a drink of water and we settled in to rest, again to be interrupted, this time by Lyle and Claire and Martha and Bill. Martha and Bill had come in to say good bye; I left the room to allow them privacy. I had already told Martha how happy I was to meet her, being my friend's sister, and how nice it had been to also meet James. She did not trust or like me, I felt, and I was glad when she left. Claire told me this was only the beginning. I had told Claire I want only what is best for my friend—what she wants, in life and for services after her death.

Kristin and Reid came in. I left them alone with Jean. I reentered after a while, and Jean motioned for me to stay. Kristin wept and I put my arm around her and told her we could talk later, if she liked. And later we did talk as Jean slept. I told Kristin that I loved her mother very much, that I had stayed home from Bermuda for very different reasons than she would have, that going away was okay for her, and not to be compared with my staying. I had to coordinate Jean's care and I wanted and needed to be here now; and it was good for her to go away with her father and brother as she had done and to continue with her life. I told how I had promised her mother 5 years ago that she would not be alone, no matter what happened. "You will never journey alone," I would always say to her. I tried to assure Kristin that her mom was well cared for and she could go to school now, if she chose, as well. She said she wanted to go, but did not want to go and have to come right back home. I said she could try it. I asked if she was able to function on vacation and she said she was okay. She cried only an hour each night. I said she could plan to come home on the weekend, but that ultimately it was her decision whether she go to school as scheduled or stay home. But I wanted her to be reassured that her mom was loved and well cared for. She went in and spent private time with Jean; Reid and I stayed out in the hall and talked. Later we joined Kristin in Jean's room. She was sitting silently crying as she stared at her mom, who was sleeping. I too sat silently staring at my friend. I told Kristin her mom was beautiful, and we both sat with tears in our eyes in total silence for a long time while Jean slept peacefully. When she woke up, intermittently, we would give her water, change her position, and hope she was at ease. She was very, very tired, and I wondered if there was more going on, as she seemed a little confused, too. I spoke to her nurse and asked if blood work had been done. She said no, as there was nothing to do with the results. I said it would be nice to know though if her BUN and creatinine went up. She agreed and had an order written to draw blood.

Roger returned with a coffee for me, as I had done for him 10 hours earlier. We chatted about the day having been full of family visits and events, and I said how awkward it had been, as I am not family but feel so protective of my friend. He reminded me that he too was not family, and we mused that we could both be thrown out—her nonfamily caregivers. It was a scary feeling. After he went into Jean's room, I entered to say good-bye to her. I hugged her gently, and she held me close for a long time. She was so soft and warm, and it felt so good to hold her and for her to hold me. I whispered I would be back tomorrow, and she said: "8 A.M.?" I said: "How about 7?" I told her to rest up. She watched me leave. I turned and winked and waved as her eyes said good-bye back. I spoke to the nurse at the nurse's station about Jean's bowels not moving, and that I would return in the early morning to see about the next steps toward discharge.

On the way home, I began to cry. I cried all the way to Monson. I talked to my friend and coworker, Joan Grier, as I felt so sad. She validated that I was not crazy and helped me to realize some very important things. I was loving Jean more and more each day and feeling closer each day as I was giving her more and more care. She was becoming more and more dependent on me to meet her needs, and I was responding to that by giving her more and more of me. It was only natural to feel closer to one you are so intensely caring for. She said you would want to hold her and cradle her, and that is exactly how I felt. I wanted to care for and comfort my friend completely. It was so beautiful and natural for me to do—to feed and bathe and toilet and console her. I was becoming her caretaker, and she had been training me to do it. We had become one: I could talk for her, as I knew what she wanted without her having to speak. I came to know her needs and could fulfill them as a mother does for her child. I also knew no one else could, for I had been trained by her, my master. I therefore felt protective of my charge and resented anyone interfering with my mission of care. I was the only one who could do the best job, and she knew it, too. Even when Kristin came in, and lunch was being served, Jean asked me to continue to feed her, as I sat by her on the bed. It was natural and I fed her like no one else could—I was the caregiver, and Kristin was her daughter. Jean and I had become a unit and I realized that to love her and respond to her needs more and more each day was natural and the way it must be: no one would be able to interrupt or understand, just as no one else can understand the tie between mother and infant. Soon Jean and I would no longer have to talk. I would just know what I must do to meet her needs. She needed to rest and I was the one who could provide it by being one with her during her transition from life to death. I would be charged with accompanying her toward that tunnel peacefully and beautifully, until she would need me no more. At that moment, I would be able to let go and deliver my friend as she relinquished life. I was not afraid, but felt strength and certainty that we would move on with our journey in peace and in love.

MONDAY, AUGUST 23

I arrived at 6:45 A.M. to find Jean asleep and Roger also, in the chair by her bed. Once he woke, he and I exchanged hellos, and I gave him a hot coffee I had brought for him. I walked him to the elevator, and as he was about to leave, we met Dr. Rayner coming to the floor to make rounds. Dr. Rayner agreed that Jean could go home, as she so desperately wanted to do. Dr. Rayner continued to offer Roger hope that radiation might help but agreed that dialysis made no sense. Dr. Rayner saw Jean, and she continued to convince him that she was ready to go home, and that was where she belonged. I watched as she mustered all her strength to plead her case for discharge, and she succeeded.

Before any nurses or Dr. Rayner came to check on her, she had vomited and convinced Roger to flush it before anyone could see. She knew she was going to die, though no doctor would openly admit it to her. She had told me that Dr. Rayner had a problem with dying patients, and I could see it clearly. This was very difficult for him as the provider who is supposed to support life. I sat by Jean's side most of the morning, protecting her from intruders—aides, housekeepers, flower deliverers—so that she could sleep. At 11:30 A.M., she went down for radiation as scheduled; at 1:30 P.M., she was discharged and went home. I had made all the arrangements, and the ambulance arrived on time to take her home. It was a glorious departure. Jean was going home in full force: no good-byes or forced conversations, just "Out of here!"

When she got to Ashford, she was welcomed by her whole family as a hero returning from battle. She was securely placed in her own bed in her own home and fell into a sound sleep—the first good sleep since her hospital admission. I stayed the night for the first time; I wanted to be near her and watch over her, as she was very lethargic. I sat in her recliner chair and kept a watchful eye all night long.

AUGUST 24

I awoke at 6 A.M. after lightly dozing and felt relieved that she had slept peacefully through the night. She continued to be tired all day, slipping in and out of sleep. At one point, though, she sat up in bed and ate a big bowl of oatmeal. Feeding was more difficult than usual, and she said, "We have to have the same goals." I knew she meant we needed to be more corrodinated in our effort. I commented that we worked together well for the most part. In fact, I was amazed at how well we did work together on most accounts and silently thought about all we had done as a team. In the late morning, I called Kristin in to the bedroom to sit with us. We had talked at length the night before; I had told her about her mother's and my relationship the past 6 years and how it had all evolved to the present. Kristin talked about her trials and tribulations during her adolescence, the conflicts with her mom over some of her adolescent behavior, which had led to her mom sending her away to a private boarding school in New Jersey to complete her high school education. She talked about how she had learned so much from her mother and how the "good" had won out. We talked about her going back to college on schedule and how difficult that decision was. Kristin is a beautiful, vibrant girl who cries easily and enjoys talking about her mom and all that the two of them have been through together, and I know she enjoyed talking to me about it all. I suggested that we would be needing each other, and that we must stay connected. She said Claire had told her to tell her mom she loved her and to ask her any questions she may want answered. Kristin said it was strange, because she had certainly already told her mom she loved her. She spoke about fearing that her mom was going to die soon, and she would get to school only to have to come right back home. She was wanting to know when her mom would die. She was trying to prepare herself and trying to make the best decisions and use the best judgment about whether to be here or at school.

So when I called Kristin in to sit with Jean and me, we sat one on either side of her, and I proceeded to tell Jean how Kristin and I had talked the night before, and that I felt that Kristin had her feet firmly planted on the ground and would be okay. I told her she could be very proud to have raised such a beautiful daughter. She looked at me and told me I should be proud too of having raised two fine children; she had seen me through their adolescence and been such a support as I followed in her footsteps trying to make difficult decisions around the crises of kids growing up. It was good for the three of us to sit and talk. I wanted Jean to know that she had done well in connecting Kristin and me and she need not worry about her daughter being alone. We then listened to a Judy Collins lullabye tape that Jean loved. It's a beautiful and soothing tape. Jean closed her eyes as she listened and mouthed the words "and if I die before I wake" and other lullabyes that Judy Collins sang so peacefully. She had a soft smile on her face and looked at peace. Kristin and I sat silently, one on either side of Jean. We each held one of her hands, and we were all connected. Jean silently sang. Kristin and I listened as tears flowed down our cheeks. Jean held my hand so tightly; she opened her eyes and looked at Kristin with love and understanding, and then she did the same toward me. It was a tender moment that makes time stand still.

Once I left Jean's room, I sobbed as I realized how cruel I felt it was to move this very ill woman by ambulance every day to Hartford Hospital for radiation treatments that clearly were not making a difference. But she continued with the scheduled regime like a trooper, still looking with some bit of hope for a miracle and a cure. We made it into Hartford and back, the treatment and blood work included, in 2 hours. Once back in her bed, Jean slept very soundly, for the trip and treatment is extremely exhausting now. In the early evening, Claire made and served a lovely dinner, and we all gathered around the table for a "family" dinner, all minus Jean. It was difficult to eat heartily, and I could not help but focus on Jean's chair at the dinner table occupied by someone else. We talked about how we had all come together and how comforting it was that we were all in agreement in how things were proceeding. Silently my thoughts were beginning to be about how much longer Jean can endure the treatments; I just wanted her to be comfortable now. I phoned the medical director where I worked and asked for more time off, as my vacation was ending, and there was no way I could return to work at this time. He asked what would change by my taking more time off. I thought it a strange question, but I knew he was really asking how much time I would need. I suggested that it would not be that long, but that I needed to continue what I had begun so long ago. The extended time off was granted.

SATURDAY, AUGUST 28

I have not had time to log in this journal since last Tuesday.

On Wednesday, Kristin left for college on schedule. The VNA nurse came; she was cold and I did not want her to continue to take care of Jean. I phoned the VNA and asked if Jean could be transferred to the hospice nurse for all her care now. With aides, the VNA nurse, the hospice nurse, the minister, friends, social worker, there was too much and the continual interruptions were so tiring for Jean. On Thursday, all visits were canceled as the lab work had revealed a hematocrit of 18.9 (very anemic), and Jean had to go to Hartford Hospital for blood transfusions. She had been phoned by the radiation nurse who asked her if she wanted the transfusions, and Jean had said yes without hesitation. This illustrated to me Jean wanted to get better and held on to hope for improvement in her condition. We went for the transfusions. By the time she was receiving the second pint of blood, I was amazed to see her color dramatically improve, and she actually awoke from her previously lethargic state. I sat with her through the whole transfusion process, fed her, helped her turn, sponged her face when a slight fever developed. Dr. Rayner came in, and he commented again that he hoped the radiation would help her situation.

On Friday, the home health aide came and I supervised this poor aide's bathing technique. I helped Jean with her mouth care, such an important part of her care, about which she is and always has been most diligent. Jean explained her complete process for mouth care, as she was preparing me, I suspected, for when she could no longer participate as actively, and I would have to take over. As more and more people like the aide were becoming involved in Jean's care, part of me didn't like it, because I was fussy about everything being done perfectly and feeling no one was living up to expectations; on the other hand, I knew it was good to have more resources in place. I welcomed the hospice nurse outside the house when I heard her arrive. I wanted her to know that there had not been much talk in the house about "hospice," as that correlates with terminal, and treatment was still being done. She understood and came inside to talk with Roger and me. It felt like she stayed too long, but she was very nice and it was good to have her as part of the team. As more people were becoming involved, Jean and I agreed we were going to have to limit people to doing their task and then leaving, as the tendency was for people to stay too long at times, and we didn't need it, as we had most things under control and Jean tired so easily. It is hard to understand how tiring everything is; even simple conversation, looking, listening, smiling, moving takes considerable energy, when there is so little to begin with. We agreed that too many resources can be as much a problem as no resources; there has to be a balance.

Jean told me to take the weekend off, as if I were someone on duty. She made me smile, as if I could go without seeing her for 2 days. Saturday, I went over to Ashford later in the day and brought dinner for a change. Jean actually sat out in the living room, and we ate shrimp cocktails together. It was wonderful. She tired rather quickly, and we moved her back to her bed. She talked to me about asking Dr. Rayner if radiation was really helping. I knew she was worried. I asked her if she felt it was making a difference. She said that she had a chronic condition and that this was a close call. I could see she was still hopeful she could possibly survive. She even walked a few steps with the walker and was pushing hard with all her strength to get better. The transfusions had helped her energy level momentarily, and she was using the momentum to push on. In the evening, she developed heartburn, which is not usual for her. I wondered if the cancer was affecting her digestive tract. Her urine output continued to be tinged pink. There were so many things not right. I was afraid of what was inside her, of the cancer taking over her body. But she did look better since the transfusion. Monday would be an important day, and she would hopefully talk with Dr. Carlson, the radiologist, and Dr. Rayner, her oncologist.

THURSDAY, SEPTEMBER 2

There has been little time to write—always something to do. I came over Sunday morning. The plan was for Claire and Lyle to take Roger out of the house for a while: to get him out for a while and to allow for Lee and Daren to visit with Jean privately. But Roger refused to go, so Claire and Lyle went themselves; I stayed with Roger. While waiting for Lee and Daren, Jean was visited by her minister, Jan, and a church deacon, who brought flowers from the parishioners. They had a short visit, and Jean was pleased that they stopped by. When Lee and Daren arrived, they checked with us as to how things were going and went in to see Jean. Roger went downstairs to his workshop retreat, and I sat out in the living room, lest Jean need anything. Halfway into their visit, she called me into her room to visit as well. We looked at family picture albums of when the children were very young. It was refreshing to look back at the pictures of the good old days, and to listen to Lee and Jean talk about them; only the good was remembered. They enjoyed sharing the memories of so long ago, down to every detail. I offered Lee coffee and got fresh ice water for Jean. I then went back into the living room to join Roger. He had gotten out his family photo albums, and he showed me pictures of himself many years ago in the army. After their visit with Jean, Lee and Daren joined Roger and me in the dining room. Lee and Roger cordially shook hands, and Lee and Daren hugged me. We talked briefly. Lee was searching for understanding of how things really were. He was pleased to hear that Jan had been by. He and Jean had attended that church long ago, and she and Roger are now members.

Earlier, I had spoken with Jan at length, at Claire's suggestion, to apprise her of different family members wanting to control the "memorial service" and that not all were in agreement with Jean's desires. I expressed my own concern that there was so much talk about the memorial, rather than people facing current life issues. Such an avoidance of current pain and sadness confused me. We talked a long while. I asked her if she ever prayed with Jean when she visited; she said Jean had not made any such overtures yet, that for now they were talking, and Jean was telling her what was important to her in the memorial service. I asked that if they did offer any prayers, that I be involved, too. She said, "Of course." I am not a praying person and never attend religious services, but I wanted to be a part of anything spiritual right now, as I was feeling a need to participate in what was happening. I also knew I was going to need Jan's spiritual guidance and support and outlook in the future, and I was making an anticipatory connection with the minister. She was easy to talk to. I explained where I was coming from honestly, and she understood. I already felt her support.

I left for home before dinner this day to allow for the family to have time together alone. Monday was going to be tense, as Dr. Carlson would be returning from a vacation, and Jean was planning to talk with him about her progress.

Monday, August 30, 1993: The ambulance did not show up on schedule. There had been a major mess-up in scheduling. After numerous phone calls to the ambulance company, to the insurance company, to Hartford Hospital radiology department, and to Dr. Carlson, we were finally picked up by the ambulance at 4 P.M., 2 hours late for Jean's radiation appointment. I had made arrangements with everyone at Hartford Hospital to wait for us, so Jean could have her treatment and, especially, so she could see Dr. Carlson, who was extremely important to her and had been away for the past week. Dr. Carlson spoke with us briefly and then went in to see Jean. She had become ill with chills and vomiting while waiting. He ordered a shot of Compazine and proceeded to tell her the nodes were shrinking, that the radiation was working—that we should continue. Jean attributed the nausea and vomiting to anxiety with the delayed ambulance and anticipation of seeing Dr. Carlson with a progress report. On the way home from the hospital, she slept. Roger sat up front with the ambulance driver—this was his first trip in the ambulance with us.

When we arrived home, we found Claire and Lyle had prepared smelts for dinner; they were absolutely delicious. All through the meal, I thought about Jean telling me how she and Roger and Lyle and Claire used to go smelting every year and the wonderful times they had. She had been surprised that I had never tasted smelts, and now as I ate them, and remembered her tales of their times together, I felt sad, as she lay sleeping in her hospital bed in the room down the hall. I felt such a mix of emotions as I sat in her seat eating one of her favorite dinners, while my poor friend slept.

Tuesday, August 31, 1993: When I arrived at the house, Claire and Lyle left for South Carolina: hurricaine Emily was hitting the state, and they needed to get home to secure their property. We were suddenly on our own. The quiet was refreshing, but I would certainly miss their support. Roger made a turkey casserole, and Jean sat in her recliner in the living room as Roger and I sat at the dining room table eating dinner. I felt extremely uncomfortable at the table with Roger, as Jean sat off and away. I felt awkward and trapped as I wondered what she thought, if anything, of all this. Then she suddenly became very ill with vomiting and diarrhea. We all three worked together to get her to the bathroom, but she was so ill. I felt helpless and so angry: this just wasn't fair. As humiliating as such a situation could be, she maintained her dignity and control, directing Roger and me to do this and that to get her needs met. She handled a horrendous situation beautifully. She never cried or yelled or gave up; she just handled what was delivered to her with such emotional strength and determination, though she was exhausted and very ill. She could accept whatever was, under the most adverse conditions, and go on. She never apologized or appeared embarrassed, but did what needed to be done to handle an ugly situation. She was an inspiration, so beautiful, even when so ill. We put her to bed finally after an ordeal I hoped would never have to be repeated. We were all exhausted; I was in awe of my friend, as always.

On Wednesday, I arrived at the house later than usual. Roger had decided to take the day off. The home health aide, the VNA nurse, and the minister all came by. James, Jean's brother, phoned the house in a panic and said to Roger, "I need to speak to Jean." He had to tell her he loved her. He spoke to her as she received her bed bath, and told her he loved her very much. While Jean was telling me what he said after she hung up from their conversation, I flashed back to a Sunday one month ago when I too had felt a compulsion to see her and drove from one friend's home 60 miles away to hers just to see and be with her. I understood the urgency that James felt.

Roger ran some errands. He had decided not to go to Hartford Hospital with us today for blood test results. He was getting weary. I stayed with Jean and she slept until 1:45 P.M. She awoke and was feeling nauseated. I helped her to the commode and then to the wheelchair to get her into the living room to await the ambulance. I cleaned the commode, emptied Jean's catheter and measured urinary output, got the ice water bottle ready, got her special lip gloss for very dry lips and mouth, got the right matching robe, turban, and slippers, and was all ready for the ambulance when it arrived. In the ambulance, Jean responded, "It only takes competence." Then I said, "Who needs four people anyway?" We smiled with each other. I even brought the emesis basin, as my friend was just not feeling well today. After radiation, I asked Dr. Carlson to give us the blood test results. They were not ready, but as he talked to Jean, she became ill and vomited. She was so sick—her nose was red, her face flushed, her eyes half-closed; I looked at him, longing for her to be given some relief. He ordered Compazine and a nurse gave her the shot. On the way home, she held her side with her hand. The jostling from the ambulance ride was uncomfortable as never before, but she never complained. Over the bumps, I held her side for her to support where the pain was, as she held tissues and the emesis basin. Once home, she was bounced on the stretcher as the drivers carried her up the steps to the house, and as soon as the ambulance left, she began to vomit. I held her weak head as she sat in the wheelchair; I wrapped my arms around her with my head next to hers, and she lay her head on mine. She never complained, but she was so ill and weak. We gave her Compazine by mouth and helped her to bed at 7:30 P.M. I left shortly thereafter for home, and I worried. I had called Dr. Carlson, and he agreed to cancel radiation for the next 5 days.

Thursday, I arrived early in the morning so that Roger could go to work for a few hours. Jean had had an anxiety attack in the bathroom and Roger had given her Ativan. With the Compazine, it really sedated her. We did not get her up until early evening. But she was confused after her long sedated sleep, which left her with no concept of time; the break in her routine—no trip to Hartford Hospital, which she had consistently done for the past 2 1/2 weeks—further added to her confusion. I explained over and over to her about her sleepiness and loss of the concept of time gently, trying to orient her without making her feel undignified or any more confused. By 9 P.M., she was back in bed. Roger and I could not eat dinner that night; we were unable to eat the evening before as well. Jean was also having bladder spasms, continually insisting she had to void, even though she had a catheter in place. She would demand to sit on the commode, and we would help her on repeatedly, trying to balance her not getting agitated with feeling some sense of control over what she wanted to do. I called the hospice nurse for some advice on how to handle the problem. I needed help and reassurance, and I got it from this nurse who had experience with these kinds of situations. I had tested out a resource for the first time, and I was offered assistance; it was good to know that the resource was available and came through. I left for home once Jean was settled for the night; again I was worried.

Friday morning, I arrived early again to find that Jean and Roger had fallen the night before (my unspoken fear, given Roger's back problem and unsteadiness on his feet at times and his fatigue). She had tried to get to the commode by herself; her weakened, numb right leg betrayed her, and she fell. Roger, in trying to help her, fell as well. Neither had been injured, but this was reason for major concern. The aide came and gave her a bed bath, and the nurse came to change her Hickman catheter dressing (changed three times a week); after these prodecures, Jean was totally exhausted, and slept in long naps as I sat by her. Roger had gone to work. Lee came to visit. I explained to him how exhausted she was, and he agreed to a short visit. As he was leaving, he said to me, "The radiation may get it in one place, but the lymphoma will grow somewhere else." His implication was, "What's the use?" He said I was a special friend, and I replied that she was a special friend. He commented we would all have to go out for a drink when this was all over, and I commented I would do my own therapy. I found his comment peculiar, and my response was a bit strange, too, but we were all weary, worried, and confused by all that was happening so quickly, I expect. I was finding people's reactions odd: Jean's sister and brother-in-law were most concerned about the memorial service, and now Lee was acting like Jean should "die, and get it over with." I was feeling that Roger and I were the only ones alive with Jean in the current time frame. I can't understand the lack of sensitivity of those family members close to Jean, as she is so sensitive and compassionate. Yet who am I to judge? I am not family, and people react differently. Maybe those who are the closest have the most difficult time being the closest as death nears. Maybe I am the fortunate one to be able to be with Jean in the current moment, as I have not known her all my life and do not have all the memories that her family members have. I am not to judge the others, but I still found the reactions and comments peculiar. I kept my thoughts to myself and within this journal, but I do wonder what she hears: the comments and whispers in the living room and dining room, as she lies in her bed. I know she must be aware at times, and I wonder what she thinks. Once people leave, I am so happy to be alone in the quiet with her, where there are no whispers or comments about her or her condition. The honest quiet is comforting. I sit in the chair by her bed as she sleeps, and a tear from nowhere flows down my cheek. My heart is breaking as my friend sleeps.

Earlier in the day she had asked me for a mirror to see her hair, which she had lost completely but which was now starting to grow back faintly. I wonder how she felt when she saw the skeletal reflection of her once-beautiful self in the mirror. I know she asked for the mirror not to see her hair but to see how she looked. I had hesitated to give it to her, but she wanted to see. She looked into her grandmother's hand mirror, stared at her reflection, and said nothing, but slowly placed the mirror on her chest and closed her eyes. I said nothing, but gently removed the mirror from her grasp and put it away. I sit here now and reflect upon that moment, and wonder.

When Roger returns from work, I go home. But I return at 5:30 P.M., as Kristin is coming home for the weekend. When I return, Kristin is there, looking beautiful, very much like her mother in so many ways. I step into the bedroom to say hello to Jean and Kristin, and then leave them alone together and go to talk with Roger as I tidy up a bit around the kitchen. When Kristin leaves her mother, she and I go out onto the deck. She asks me to talk with her brother Daren, as she believes he is confused. She says Roger tells Daren his mom will live; their father is telling him his mom will die in a matter of days. I agree I will talk with Daren; it is good to know that Kristin trusts me and feels she can ask me to talk to her brother, who is worrying her. I just hope I can live up to her expectations. We go on to talk about all the different perspectives on the situation, and I say, "There is no negative or positive, but only what is." Roger keeps talking about always being positive, and it gets confusing, because the inference is that to contemplate death at all is negative. And that just is not the case: facing death can also be positive; holding on to false hope can be negative. But Roger does not understand this, and it makes it difficult for Kristin and Daren. It is difficult to know how to intervene, but Kristin and I try to talk it out, as I want her to face reality and not feel that in so doing, she is being negative. As for Roger, I have tried to talk with him, but he is unable to face the possibility of death at this time and must hold on to undying hope. As we talk, Roger prepares Kristin's favorite dinner, macaroni and cheese. He is clearly under stress and snaps at Kristin about something, and she cries easily. I tell her he is on edge. She sobs that he has a terrible life, that he is never happy. I feel sorry for Kristin; she is so young and having to deal with so much. We get Jean to come out for dinner.

The night before, I had had Jean sit at the table for the first time in her wheelchair on a trial basis, in preparation for tonight's dinner with Kristin at home. She comes out and we get her in the wheelchair to the table. She is weakened by nausea and a tedious trip to the commode before coming out, but she makes a gallant effort. She has a Compazine tablet on her plate, and a glass of Suplena supplement, as Kristin serves the rest of us macaroni and cheese; it is so pathetic. I feel so sorry but, sickeningly, I also see the humor. My sense of humor has deteriorated, but I expect it is a defense against the opposite emotion of wretched sadness. And then, unexpectedly, Jean says with tremendous sarcasm, "Invite a friend for dinner. We are having Compazine, followed by Suplena and applesauce. Throw in good nursing care mixed up with friendship and love." She is angry. She looks me straight in the eye as she says this, not at all lovingly, but with cold anger. I think to myself, "Sometimes I think she despises me." And I realize how awful it must be for her to see me healthy and eating in her home with her family while she is so ill and becoming so dependent on me at the same time. I am helpless to change this. Kristin goes on to show her mother pictures of her recent vacation with Lee and Daren. Jean looks at the pictures but continues to appear very angry. There are also pictures of Jean from some months before; Jean does not appear to want to look at them, but Kristin wants to share looking at them with her mom, and comments: "Look at my beautiful mother." She is trying so hard to make Jean feel good. Jean does not respond. I am feeling uncomfortable, but I ride it out. Kristin proceeds to continue to control the conversation and goes on to tell me about a bump on Lee's forehead. Jean pipes in, "Great conversation piece. Look, my bump is bigger than your bump. And it's growing inside me and it's killing me." She laughs sarcastically. I blurt out, "That's not funny, Jean." She retorts, "But you have to have humor." But she is not laughing. I put my hand on her shoulder and simply say, "I do love you, dear heart." I want her to stop this torture. Kristin continues to show pictures. Suddenly Jean must make a run to the bathroom—diarrhea. We return her to the table, and she is more tired yet but continues in her gallant effort to be at the table with her family for just a little while longer. Fnally, she decides to go to bed. Kristin takes her into her bedroom. After a while I go in to say goodnight. It is good to have Kristin home with her mother; this is such an important time. I kiss Jean and tell her I love her dearly, that I will not be there tomorrow. I decide to skip a day for the first time in 4 weeks, but Kristin is home and she and her mom need time together, and Kristin can care for her. I tell her I will miss her though, but will see her Sunday. I tell her to be good for her daughter, and to enjoy. She says thank you for everything, and I know she means it, despite her angry comments earlier. I wish I could stay with her forever. Roger hugs me good-bye in the hallway as I prepare to leave, and I watch her watch him. I wonder what she is thinking. I wave good-bye to her. It is so hard to leave, knowing I won't be back for 2 days; but my beeper is on should they need me.

Saturday, September 4: I call in the morning to check in. Jean had been up during the night to the commode a number of times, and she had been vomiting. I want desperately to go over, but I strongly feel this family needs to be together and in control. I call in the evening. She was up a good part of the day, and Kristin spent a lot of good time with her, though she was continuing to vomit. Roger gave her a shot of Compazine. I was worried about dehydration now. Kristin said the catheter tubing may be clogged. I suggest we can call the hospice nurse. I tell Roger I will begin to share night duty as the days go by. He is asking for help now during the day as well. I will call the hospice nurse on Monday. Tomorrow, Sunday, I will go over to help with a Sunday bath before the minister comes.

SEPTEMBER 22, 1993

I haven't written since September 4. So much has happened.

Sunday, September 5, I went over to Ashford in the morning, as planned. I was so anxious to see my friend after skipping a Saturday visit. I am worried. Jean is tired and weak, but clearly happy to see me by the welcoming and warm look in her eyes. I proceed to give her a bath for the first time. I give a nice full bath, slowly and deliberately, comfortingly, and she relaxes throughout. It is a lovely day, and the sun shines in warmly through mostly closed curtains. I suggest as I bathe her that maybe she can go outside for 5 minutes later today, just to smell the air—it is such a lovely sunny summer day, and I am knowing that her opportunities to experience life are getting limited. Kristin prepares to go back to school, packing her things in her bedroom next door. Jean dozes on and off during and after her bath. I have Kristin come in to Jean's room so we can all three talk, and I tell Jean once again what a wonderful daughter she has, mature and with a good head, and how Kristin acknowledged to me that "Mom had done right in sending me off to boarding school." I am trying to tie up loose ends for them both. Jan, Jean's minister, arrives at the house after Sunday services at the church. I leave them alone. Jean calls me in for a prayer service and communion. I feel privileged, sinner that I am, but I am feeling a need to be spiritually involved at this time. Kristin and Roger are invited in, too, but they refuse; I am surprised Kristin does not come in. There is no way I would miss this moment; I feel I need a connection to something greater than life and me, a connection to Jean and to this minister and all that she may have to offer. I sit with Jean, at her left side, and Jan sits to her right. Jan prepares the communion bread and wine. I actually partake of the ceremony. Jean eats her piece of bread (only piece of solid food in days, I think) and insists I drink her wine, as she is unable, and comments she will drink Carnation Instant Breakfast instead. I chuckle to myself, and my eye twinkles at Jean. I eat my bread and drink two wines. We then all three hold hands and recite the Lord's Prayer together so beautifully. I am raised to a level of peace, and Jean dozes off as we finish. We continue to hold hands, and then Jan and I look at each other and slowly release our hands, as I continue to hold Jean's hand. I wish this moment would last forever, and it does.

Jan picks up her wares to leave, and I follow her out to her car. We talk a long while about religion, about Jean being weaker, about the memorial service, about how I want to focus on now rather than who will say what for how long at the service. Jan asks me who I talk to and how I will get through this. I tell her I am forming my connection now with her in preparation.

In the afternoon, Daren comes over. He is quiet, and I encourage him to sit with his mom. He tends to want to let me stay in the room with her, and he sits in the living room. He joins her and she dozes in and out of sleep. He tells me I can sit with her soon when he tires. He seems uneasy.

Jean does not get up today. She never makes it to the living room, let alone to the outside fresh air, as I had earlier suggested. She has some more Carnation Instant Breakfast, and after her night care and retirement for the night, I leave for home.

Monday, September 5, Labor Day: I return early. No home health aide or RN visits today; it is a holiday. Jean is getting more and more sleepy. She's hardly responding to Roger or me when we talk to her now. I am getting very worried. I put in calls to Dr. Carlson and Dr. Rayner; both answering services inform me that neither is on call this holiday weekend. I speak to the covering doctors and ask them to contact Drs. Carlson and Rayner. Dr. Carlson finally returns my call. I describe the situation and Jean's symptoms: low fever, unresponsive, decreased intake and output. I ask if he ever does a home visit, and I expect he senses my desperation. He takes the directions to Jean's house from Hartford, 40 miles away, and says without hesitation that he will be out. I am so relieved and impressed with his agreeing to make a house call 40 miles away on a holiday.

On Sunday, I had spoken alone with Daren as to how he saw things, what he wanted for his mom, how he felt about continued treatment. He stated he felt his mom should not be put through anymore, that he and Kristin had talked and that they had said their good-byes. They both felt it was significant that Jean had not responded when Kristin said, as she was leaving for school, "I will see you in 2 weeks." I also felt it was significant that Jean had pulled all her strength together to be with Kristin on this past weekend, and that now, within hours of Kristin leaving, she had weakened considerably. I wanted Dr. Carlson to see Jean's status for himself so we could all come to consensus on the current plan of action. Jean was scheduled to resume radiation tomorrow. How could she even withstand the drive in, let alone transfers from bed to stretcher?

When he arrived, Dr. Carlson went in to see Jean. From a very sound sleep, she actually brightened to see him and smiled and said glowingly, "You're here? How did you get here?" She tried with all her last bit of energy to carry on a normal conversation, before falling back into sound slumber within a minute or two. It was amazing how she rallied for the last time to that extent. She was so happy to see her Dr. Carlson, to whose care she had been entrusted for so many years. It was equally as phenomenal how her energy dwindled so quickly and she again became very lethargic after a brief moment of high enthusiasm. Dr. Carlson came out and spoke with Roger and me and suggested we could hospitalize Jean, start intravenous fluids, hydrate her, do blood cultures, start antibiotics, and so forth. I said bluntly, "What for? What would it do?" He said, "Prolong her life for another week or two." I reiterated to him what she had said so many times to me over the past few months that she "wanted to die sooner rather than later." I told him how she had asked me for help with the decision, and that she needed help with the decision now. He listened and he began to finally hear. He said he would talk with Jean and ask her what she wanted. When he asked her what she wanted, she did not respond. He felt that this lack of response was her answer not to continue. She had responded to him minutes before, and this lack of response was significant, he felt. As he turned to leave her room, she said to him from behind, "Don't eat too many chocolate chip cookies on the way home!" They had had a long-standing joke about his chocolate chip cookies. She was so alert in so many ways, and yet unresponsive almost at the same time. Roger, Dr. Carlson, and I talked some more out in the dining room and agreed it was time to do what Jean wanted. As I interpreted it, Dr. Carlson finally gave Jean the okay, "the permission to die at home." I was happy. I was sad. I was scared. I was responsible. I admired Dr. Carlson. We discussed pain management, and he left it up to Roger and me to use the Duragesic patch or morphine by injection, as needed. We could call him anytime. I thanked him. Roger and I were on our own. I stayed the night in the recliner chair in Jean's room and kept a watchful eye on her as she slept.

Tuesday, September 6: I called the VNA and Paula, the hospice nurse, came over. We changed the Hickman dressing and she checked the urinary catheter. One night the catheter had come out and I had to call the VNA nurse in the middle of the night to reinsert a new one. Paula and I prepared the bed with a drawsheet. We cut a nightgown up the back for easy placement over Jean, so we would not have to make her uncomfortable if we had to change it, for any movement now was painful and she was essentially unresponsive. We placed Chux pads under her. I felt strange, for we were really doing those last-step, end-stage procedures to make someone as comfortable and tidy as possible—and that someone was Jean. We were so methodical as we worked as a nurse team now. My dear friend was completely bedridden and mostly unconscious. The home health aide now annoyed me, as I felt she was insensitive to the real situation; of course, I was probably supersensitive myself, as the reality of the seriousness of the situation was becoming painfully clear. Nonetheless, we asked her not to come anymore. I would stay and care for Jean totally now, with Roger. That felt most comfortable and right. James, Jean's brother, phoned; I explained to him that Jean might not respond but that I would put the phone to her ear for him to speak to her. I told Jean that James was on the line and I would put the phone to her ear. She did not respond as I spoke, but I put the phone to her ear anyway. I will never know how she, from an unconscious state, brightened, actually opened her eyes, and mouthed the words silently, "I love you"—her last words to James.

Wednesday, September 8: We no longer force fluids; we do mouth care. We turn her head as she vomits small amounts of bile. We no longer change her position. We provide comfort as best we can. Roger gives her morphine shots every 4 to 6 hours. I talk to Jean constantly and encourage her to "go easy" and to "let go," that "Kristin and Daren and Roger are okay." I had been telling her about the three of them being okay now for days. I had been assuring her all was well, she had done a good job, had been a wonderful mother, nurse, lover, and friend. I believe she heard me, as she would partly smile at times and show expression on her face as I talked soothingly and reassuringly to her. I told her as well how much I loved her and all she had meant to me. In the late night hours, I suddenly realized I had not told her something. I cried and said I was very sad, that I would miss her, but that I, too, would be okay, and she could leave us all now. That night I did not sit in the recliner as I had been doing the previous two nights. I sat in a straightback chair right next to her bed and softly held her hand. Soon I found I was sitting on the floor next to her bed, so I could rest my aching back and lower my head as I lightly dozed. Suddenly, I was up on my feet with a start and felt totally awake and alert. It was nearly 4 A.M., and I knew Jean could have another shot, which Roger was adamant about her getting on schedule. I did not want to give it, for I could see her respirations were slower, and I knew the morphine could depress them even more. I had been counting her respirations all night—they were down to only five per minute at times, and she was having apneic spells [breathing stops] regularly. I went to draw the morphine into the syringe and call Roger, as he wanted to give it to her. He wouldn't waken. I awoke his friend who had come over around midnight to be with Roger this night, and she continued to try to wake Roger, asleep in the living room recliner. I returned to Jean's room. Her respirations were now light, regular, and unlabored, and there was something different about the peaceful, light way she was breathing. She was relaxed, and I knew she was about to die. I held her hand. Roger came in. He kissed her and hugged her and proceeded to place the blood pressure cuff on her arm. I motioned "no" and he stopped. She was dying. I held her hand and felt her last pulse beat. She was so beautiful, and finally at rest.

We cried. I called the hospice nurse, and then went and sat with my beloved friend for the last time. I couldn't leave her. I wiped her eyes. I held her hand some more. I covered her snuggly with her blanket. I placed her pink turban on her head, as she would want it. She was still there and still my friend for whom I was caring. I stayed until the nurse came, and then stayed on until the undertaker came. My heart broke as they took her away; I stood in the driveway, the early light of dawn outlining the van as it slowly left the yard and drove down the quiet street. I called everyone who needed to know: James, Martha, Kristin's school therapist who would tell Kristin, Lee, Jean's best friends, Dr. Carlson, Dr. Rayner, everyone. I would cry for days.

My dearest friend died September 9, 1993, at 4:30 A.M., after a courageous 9-year struggle with non-Hodgkin's lymphoma. I spent most of my time the next few days in her room, or in her office with all her books and memorabilia. Roger's family came: brother, sister, son, daughter, nieces and nephews. Their noise annoyed me, but their presence was such a comfort for Roger and that was most important, for his loss was the greatest. I wanted only to be quietly with Jean's belongings. I was glad Roger had his family, and that I had the comfort of being with Jean's things, in her bedroom where she died, in her office. Daren, Lee, and Reid left to go get Kristin in Pennsylvania and bring her home. When she arrived at the house, she hugged Roger for a very long time, and then me. It was so difficult for her, for she had not been there the past few days, and she was stunned: the house was full of people, but not her mom.

I went to see Jan, the minister, the next day, Friday, as I wanted to talk about the planned memorial service, and to say I would like to say a few words as well, if appropriate. I wanted to be sure that the service was going to be the way Jean so desperately wanted; it was something she had planned for a long time: what hymms and psalms, the people she wanted to speak. Jan assured me she had spoken to everyone, as everyone had their own ideas: Jean's sister and her brother-in-law, who would read parts of the scripture; Lee, who had been a part of this congregation with Jean for years when they were married; Claire, who had wanted Jan to be aware of everybody's ideas, which were sometimes in conflict; and me, who simply wanted it all to be the way Jean wanted it. Jan was great; she had listened to everyone, but especially to Jean, and had the service planned just the way Jean wanted it. She reassured me, and I was grateful. I had never realized all that went into the planning of a memorial service, but Jan was clearly in charge, and had everyone's number, and was dealing with each person's need to grieve and be part of the service in individual ways. But her prime concern was to tailor the service to Jean's plan. She was good, and I felt reassured that Jean's desires would be fulfilled. Jean had planned everything, even had talked about a Saturday service so people could come and not have to miss work, and sure enough she died on a Thursday and the service would be "as planned," on a Saturday.

Saturday, September 11: A beautiful memorial service on a sunny day in late summer in a beautiful church with over 200 people in attendance—a lovely service, just as Jean had planned. Jan spoke beautiful words about Jean, her character, her love of family and friends, her concern for all of us, and her concern as expressed to Jan right up to the end for Roger and me as we cared for her in the last days of her life. Bill read from the scripture and spoke about Jean's wonderful life. James spoke about his beloved sister and her love for family, friends, and the people she worked with; about her character and attributes, her achievements and accomplishments in a full, though short, life.

I spoke next, briefly, about the last few weeks of Jean's life and what we talked about and I shared with the congregation comforting words about death I would read to get me through the very sad times the last few weeks:

Death does bring changes and adjustments for those left behind. The warmth and associations of former days are gone. The silence, the finality, the incommunicability disturb. But for the one who has triumphed, there is rejoicing. Sorrow is centered more on self than on the deceased. One grieves, yet we would not want our grief taken from us, even if it could be, for our love is wrapped up with our grief. Grief is the price we pay for love. "Love is eternal. Death is a horizon, and the horizon is only the limit of our sight." It has been said, "Death is not extinguishing the light, but putting out the lamp because the dawn has come."

I went on to say: "Just before dawn on September 9, Jean died and triumphed, and for her we should rejoice as we celebrate her remarkable and distinguished life."

Following me, Charlie, the former CEO of the insurance company Jean and I worked for, read an original prayer. He had always had a special relationship with Jean, and immediately upon my notifying him of Jean's death, he mailed his prayer he had written for her days before, with regret that she had not received it before her death. After reading the very beautiful prayer, I contacted him and asked if I might read it at the memorial service, and later decided it would be so much better if he read it himself. He agreed and was honored. As he finished reading, a bell tolled from somewhere outside (the church sits in a row of churches on the UConn campus) in perfect synchrony, totally unplanned.

After him, Ann, Jean's friend from childhood, spoke about their lives together over the years and how they had been "best friends for life." Roger's niece sang a most beautiful rendition of the hymn "How Great Thou Art," Jean's favorite. As she sang, sunshine streamed in so perfectly through the windows of the church. Everyone in attendance was very sad, but at peace. I sat next to Kristin, and next to me sat Lee and then Daren. Reid sat on the other side of Kristin. Roger did not attend the memorial service, as had already been prearranged with Jean, as he felt he just could not do it, and she accepted his decision. He spent the time with his son and his brother. I felt his absence, but understood it was his decision.

Following the service, people gathered in the building adjoining the church, and there were lots of talk and hugging, tears and quiet laughter. And then we all went our own ways. I went back to the house to see Roger, and shortly thereafter, I, too, went home. Not a day goes by that I do not play the tape of the memorial service: it is such a beautiful and inspiring service and has Jean's plan woven throughout.

Today, September 22, is the first day I did not go to see anyone at Jean's house. Today, Kristin left to return to school. Roger started medication yesterday. I miss my friend desperately and talk and pray to her all the time. She's now my guardian angel, I am sure.

OCTOBER 1, 1993

Nine more days gone by. I still cry. I carry her pictures with me. I wear her watch, which I had used to take her pulse so many times. So many people have sent me beautiful cards and notes about their love for Jean, but mostly about the gift Jean and I gave each other. People I never before connected with are now opening up in very spiritual, emotional ways to me, as I expect they see me as a last connection to Jean, whose loss they too are grieving. I cry so much; I miss her desperately. I think about all of this—what happened, what I failed to do, how I wish we had been closer years ago, how I never appreciated the fear and pain my friend lived with for 9 years; how she so desperately reached out to me years ago and I did not totally grasp the depth of her reach, the sincerity of her need. I feel I failed her then, even though the die was cast for what was to transpire these past few months, when I would give all that I could to meet her needs in the final phase of her life.

I just wish I could have one more day, one more hour, one more minute to tell her all I want to say about our friendship and love, and to comfort her one more time. Therapists say to take it slowly. Some people say the pain never goes away, that you just learn to live with it. Whatever is the case, my life is changed. I thank God for my friend, for the gift of her friendship and love, and I pray that I, too, can be a good person. On October 16, I will fly to be a guest at an annual conference on alcohol and substance abuse in Oregon, which is being dedicated to Jean's memory. I am afraid to fly and leave my son home, as he is having problems, but nothing can keep me from honoring my friend as her colleagues praise and honor her.

NOVEMBER 7, 1993

It has been nearly 2 months since Jean's death, and there is not a day that I do not think about her. I feel she is with me, and I still feel she is a part of the team at work. Her picture and name plate hang in my office, and I find comfort in their being there. I talk to her and know we still share a secret communication. I miss her so much. Others at work confide in me that they talk to her, too, and feel her presence still.

I went to Oregon, and Jean was described as a pioneer in managed alcohol and substance abuse care. I was with people from around the country who knew her, and that felt good. I wish I had been more a part of her life and we had had more mutual experiences, as I was now experiencing what was hers without her. Kristin, Roger, Daren, and I keep in touch. I go over to Ashford, but not often, as I try to get my life back in order and allow Roger to do the same. But it is such a comfort to be with Jean's family. We are very close, as Jean planned and so diligently orchestrated; whenever I think of her mastery in setting stages for the acts to follow, I smile. Kristin and I go to the church where Jean's memorial service was held whenever she is home from school. Roger keeps Jean's ashes on a table close by his bed. I tried to stop carrying around pictures and cards, but today I went and retrieved some I had put away, as I am feeling the need to have her memories with me again. For a few weeks, I did okay, but I am feeling so sad and lonely again, as Thanksgiving approaches. She always sent me such beautiful cards at Thanksgiving and always wrote personal notes on how thankful she was for me, and I can't remember if I ever even sent her a single Thanksgiving card. I took them out yesterday and read them over and over again. I will carry them around with me over this holiday. The insurance company I work for published a cookbook *From the Heart* and dedicated it to Jean; her recipe in her own handwriting is on the first page. It is heartwarming. Proceeds from the sale of the cookbooks go to the United Way. I daydream about dedicating a conference room to her memory and will present the idea in time, once our company moves to its new location.

Jan, Jean's minister, called me, and we chatted for well over an hour on the phone. I was so pleased. She offers good insights. I told her how the sadness will never leave, and she said she did not think that that was bad, because "if the sadness goes, so does the intimacy." I felt warmed by that statement. Some simple thoughts or statements can mean so much, I am finding out. Another that comforts me is "Each life is complete unto itself." In other words, it matters not how long or how short a life is. Each is its own complete entity: an infant who lives 1 minute, a man who lives 90 years. Each has its own meaning and purpose and impact. I hang on to thoughts I find comforting, and I am sure different people find their own individual comforting thoughts or statements to hang onto. I do not cry all the time now; but every now and then, the overwhelming sadness hits. My sadness now is more internal and less expressive. I continue to value solitude, and my current friendships are not as intense as they once were. My closest friend is becoming Roger, for we are the only ones who know what we have been through without even talking about it. I have been reading a lot about spirits living on after they leave their earthly bodies, about reincarnation, about life after death, and I feel hopeful. Maybe I will one day again be reunited with my friend. For now, I choose to believe I will.

Epilogue

November 1994: A year has passed since my last entry into my journal. In some respects, a year ago seems so long ago; in other ways, it seems like yesterday. When people would say, time heals, I heard but did not believe; now I understand. Time does take away the pain, and the memories do become a comfort. Sadness lingers, but with acceptance. When I was advised to take as much time as I needed to heal, I did. I also did what I wanted to help ease my sadness, like carrying Jean's picture, wearing her watch, doing little things that reminded me of her and her wonderful inspiration. I talked about her and I kept her memory very alive, as did other colleagues at work, and certainly Roger and her children and friends did the same. Keeping the memory alive is very comforting and healing. Healing is a process, and a very individual experience that varies in intensity and in time.

I ordered laminated memorial cards with Jean's picture, obituary, and the 23rd Psalm on it, and gave them out to her colleagues and friends. It is a comfort to walk around the company and see them tacked up here and there in people's workstations. And when there was turmoil at work, someone would always comment, "I wonder what Jean would say" or "How would Jean handle this problem?" She remained so much a part of the team at work. In time, we were even able to laugh about what Jean's response might have been, and at other times, we would actually take the advice we knew she would give if she were alive—a real tribute to her consistent inspiration to us all.

In May 1994, Roger planned a trip to Rockport, Massachusetts, to deliver Jean's ashes to the sea, her final wish. She had instructed Roger to throw them into the harbor where they used to go for time away together. Roger, Kristin, Reid, and I went, and we followed a program arranged by Roger. We read prayers and played the recording of "How Great Thou Art" as sung at the memorial service. Roger threw the ashes into the sea, and Kristin threw in a dozen long-stem red roses over the ashes. It was a beautiful day. Seagulls flew overhead, bells tolled, and we sat silently on the rocks and watched as the tide took the ashes away. This was Roger's memorial service, more than anyone else's, and very beautiful.

On July 15, 1994, which would have been Jean's 50th birthday, our company dedicated the Jean E. Campbell Conference Room. The dedication was arranged by Peggy Schoer and myself, another employee and friend of Jean, and a plaque with the inscribed dedication surrounded by handpainted daffodils (the flower of the cancer society) hangs on the wall in the room.

On September 9, 1994, the anniversary of Jean's death, I felt much of the sadness return, and there is something to be said for anniversaries being a difficult time. I allowed myself one week of sadness and unexpected tears once again, and I was able to remember the good and happy times as well.

It was at Thanksgiving time that I decided to collect this journal, and put it to type, so I might share it as I had promised Jean I would. It is at Thanksgiving that I reflected on how thankful I am for having known Jean, and for having been part of her life and for her having been such an important part of mine. It is now that I understand the depth of her words: "I am thankful for you," which she would say every Thanksgiving. And I say those words back to her this Thanksgiving, and every day. And, as she would say, for every day I am grateful.

CRITICAL-THINKING ACTIVITIES

1. Tease out the principles and philosophies that guided the care that Linda Trott gave her friend Jean. Do you see any similarity between her principles and those recommended by Macurdy in Chapter 2? Compare and contrast the two.

2. Do you find correspondences between the author's way of facing fear and that of Mark Nepo, described in Chapter 14?

3. How different was the discharge planning provided for Jean in this journal than that of Professor Higgins' in Chapter 11.

4. How does the way in which Jean's pain was managed differ from the management of Mr. Armstrong's pain in "An Unhappiness Factor"? From Mr. Gordon's pain in "Reconceptions"?

5. Is there a difference between the way in which Jean, her companion, and her children were guided in their experience of the health-care system and Dr. Buck's experience, as described in "Raoul"?

6. Mason's flashpoints on the experience and power of grief are relevant to all of the members of Jean's family, Jean, her chaplain, Linda Trott, the health-care professionals, and the readers of this journal. Write a paper in which you explore the effects of sorrow and grief on each. How does the experience of each interplay with the others?

7. How has the experience of Linda Trott been distilled in Professor Mason's *Gilgamesh*?

8. What would you say is the "wonderment of the journey" that Linda Trott evokes? Elaborate.

9. How do the facets of compassion that are evident between these two women resemble Mark Nepo's experience with Paul in "God, Self, and Medicine"?

10. Write an essay describing the ways in which this journal has affected you.

Afterword

I have been asked how this book came about and must say to the reader that it had its beginnings long ago. It is a book about compassion, the search for it, what it is, and how it works. In other writings I have talked about compassion as central to all inter-actions and actions in health care. It must never, in my estimation, be viewed as merely a kindly feeling of sympathy toward another who is suffering. Compassion demands far, far more from us. And it offers much more than pity.

Of course, I didn't have any inkling of what exactly I was searching for when I first became aware of a shadowy sadness. That sadness entered my life the week of my fourth birthday. My aunt had expected a baby on that same day and my parents and I had gone to visit her. Arriving at her home, I was confronted with a hushed silence. My aunt remained in her bed with the door closed and I was not allowed to go to her. I asked my mother what was wrong and I learned that the baby had been stillborn. I couldn't comprehend the full implication of that but what I did realize was that my aunt was overcome; when I actually did see her, she looked dispirited and very pale. I also learned that the death was not to be talked about. It was apparent to me that there was no little baby, and that there wasn't going to be. What I didn't learn until years later was that my aunt had been told she couldn't have another child—she had a double sorrow. (Fortunately, this proved not to be the case.)

Several years later my sadness deepened when another aunt lost her 5-month-old baby suddenly while he was sleeping. This baby I had known well, as I had been with the family part of the summer and had helped to take care of him. No one told me directly that he had died but I heard my mother scream it to my father early that morn-ing when she received the phone call. The young children were kept away from the funeral and not included in any of the discussions. I think that the adults felt that they were sparing us from the grief that they felt.

However, I did receive a measure of comfort from a conversation I overheard in my grandmother's kitchen, where all of the adults had gathered to drink coffee. The consolation came from a question my father's brother asked of my parents. "How is Jeanine taking the baby's death? She must be very upset, since she helped take care of him all summer."

I remember wanting to feel that moment of reprieve from my sadness again and wondered why I couldn't. But I also thought about it as something that my aunts needed, too. Throughout those years I helped these aunts and uncles over school vaca-tions and in the summers with their growing families and felt very close to them. At times I helped out when there was sickness as well, and it seemed natural to think of becoming a nurse. And I had known the community nurse who was called for all manners of emergencies; she always seemed to know what to do and what to say. I wanted to be in that position.

I became a nurse's aide at the community hospital at this nurse's suggestion "to see if it is what you really want." There I saw much that dismayed me. And while I could help in very pragmatic ways, I could do nothing about the real suffering I saw. I couldn't find answers to my questions. However, I figured that by the time I had completed a degree in nursing I would have the answers to some of those questions.

And to some extent I did, more pragmatically than spiritually, though a whole new set of troubling events produced more disturbing questions. I was truly disconcerted by the emotionally disturbed children that had to be hospitalized—most especially by the wish of some of those children to end their lives. Because the university hospital was a major medical center, it accepted severely injured children and I was not prepared for the painful treatments and procedures necessary for these children's survival.

I still imagined that psychology would be able to provide me with the answers that I sought. What to make of all this suffering? How can I be of any help? Who will console me, for I felt wounded, too.

My graduate education in psychiatric mental health nursing did answer some of these ponderings, but the spiritual dimension remained unanswered. This became abundantly clear when I became the clinical nurse specialist for the burn unit and the neurology service of another major medical center. The devastating losses and grief, the profound remorse experienced by certain individuals at times staggered the nurses and myself. By now the reprieve that I wanted for my aunts and myself I wanted for the nursing and medical staff and others as well.

As I continued with my graduate studies I began to find certain artists that, at last, provided insights into the workings of compassion by their very understanding of the nature of suffering. The day that I read these lines from Sophocles' *Philoctetes*:

> *Hark! 'tis the voice of one in pain,*
> *Travelling hardly, the deep strain*
> *Of human anguish, all too clear,*
> *That smites my heart, that wounds mine ear.*

I had a similar feeling of being understood that I had all those years ago when I heard my uncle through the kitchen door.

But it was Kurosawa and Tolstoy who taught me, through *Ikiru* and *The Death of Ivan Ilych*, of the utter necessity of finding meaning in one's life and for one's life. That Kurosawa's Watanabe and Tolstoy's Ivan Ilych found that meaning only through their suffering and their illness was intrinsic information. Finding Mason's *Gilgamesh* allowed me, at last, to know that my lingering sadness was a sorrow defined by others long ago that I share, just as I do the question that Ivan Ilych and Gilgamesh asked, what else is there, is there anything after all of this suffering, this loss, this sorrrow?

The day I first saw Rodin's sculpture, "The Burghers of Calais," I saw flashes of former patients, family, friends—myself, even. These six men facing the loss of their lives in order to save the starving citizens of Calais commune with all of us. Their anger, fear, resignation, despair, confusion, resentment remind me of all the levels of consciousness we function on in our daily lives and practice. And they evoke the sacrifices that we make for others so that they might have a meaningful life, and ultimately a decent death.

But however many answers and understandings were given to me over the years through education, further readings and research, the elusive factor has always been that of the personal. What can those who have been compromised and vulnerable, afflicted with sudden wounds—psychological, spiritual, and, yes, physical—tell those of us who profess to "care" for them? What can they tell us of true caring? How can they help us to become compassionate health-care professionals?

These accounts, I believe, will be read and reread for a long time to come for their value in this regard.

Jeanine Young-Mason, EdD, RN, CS, FAAN, a graduate of the University of Michigan School of Nursing, is Associate Professor of Nursing at the University of Massachusetts at Amherst, where she teaches writing seminars in nursing studies and community mental health nursing in the graduate and undergraduate programs. She is a psychiatric-mental health clinical nurse specialist with a Doctorate in Humanistic and Behavorial Studies from Boston University. Previously she was clinical instructor at Tufts New England School of Medicine and also clinical nurse specialist at Massachusetts General Hospital.

Young-Mason writes a regular column on "Nursing and the Arts" in *Clinical Nurse Specialist: Journal for Advanced Nursing Practice*. She is the author of *States of Exile: Correspondences Between Art, Literature and Nursing* (National League for Nursing, 1995), *21 Words for Nurses* (Diamond Press, 1995), and the forthcoming *Country Practice*.